THE ULTIMATE HCG Tracker

A Fun and Easy Program for Losing Weight!

Julie Vincent

ISBN: 1456485342
ISBN-13: 9781456485344

Disclaimer:

This manual is not intended to provide medical advice or to take the place of medical advice and treatment from your personal physician. Readers are advised to consult their own doctors or other qualified health professionals regarding the treatment of medical conditions.

The author shall not be held liable or responsible for any misunderstanding or misuse of the information contained in this manual or for any loss, damage, or injury caused or alleged to be caused directly or indirectly by any treatment, action, or application of any food or food source discussed in this manual.

The statements in this book have not been evaluated by the U.S. Food and Drug Administration. This information is not intended to diagnose, treat, cure, or prevent any disease.

Since 1975, the FDA has required labeling and advertising of hCG to state: hCG has not been demonstrated to be an effective adjunctive therapy in the treatment of obesity. There is no conclusive evidence that it decreases weight beyond that resulting from caloric restriction or that it decreases the hunger and discomfort associated with calorie-restricted diets.

Table of Contents

ULTIMATE HCG TRACKER
By Julie Vincent

Introduction
By Julie Vincent

Many of us spend way too much time and energy worrying about our weight. We know that if we could just lose that weight we would feel better and could then function at our optimal best. When we feel our best, we make the best contribution to families, work, communities and the world! You deserve to be that person at your best! That fabulously, happy, healthy person! No matter what size you are!

Congratulations on deciding to use the HCG Diet! You are sure to have success if you follow the diet carefully. The nice part about it is that, though it is restrictive, it is only restrictive for 3 weeks! I don't know about you, but I can do anything for 3 weeks! Don't be nervous or afraid to get started! By day two you will understand why, **your hunger will be gone!** I'm not kidding you! This diet is easy – breezy! And 3 weeks from now, you are going to feel on top of the world, twenty pounds less than you are today!

In this book the diet has been simplified for the average, everyday person to follow. This book is for many of us who don't want to learn everything about homeopathy. For those of us who are not really going to buy organic. And most of all, for all of us who need to **lose a lot of weight fast and effectively**, without wasting a lot of time!

1

So let's get started!

What is Human Chorionic Gonadotropin (HCG)?

HCG is a natural hormone which is produced in great quantities during a pregnancy. It ensures delivery of proper nutrients to the developing infant. HCG is what actuates the hypothalamus to utilize stored fat to be used as "food". It is believed that HCG resets your metabolism and safeguards your body's healthy fat and protects muscle tissue from deteriorating, which can occur while on other low calorie diets and not using HCG.

The History of HCG

In the 1950's, Dr. A.T.W. Simeons began administering small doses of HCG to obese patients to help decrease their appetite. He discovered that **this hormone could assist dieters to lose weight and could curb one's appetite tremendously!** Since then, HCG has continued to gain popularity as a successful, natural supplement for diet and weight loss. For complete understanding of how this diet works, you can view Dr. Simeons' HCG Manuscript at www.myHCGsource.com.

What is Homeopathy?

Understanding how Homeopathy works is not a requirement to losing weight on this diet. Many people choose Homeopathic remedies as an alternative to conventional medicine. In brief, homeopathic remedies are prepared by a series of dilutions which is done by shaking, or forcefully striking after each dilution.
Homeopathy works on the principle that extreme dilution enhances the curative properties of a substance, while eliminating any possible side effects. This is just the reverse of conventional drug philosophy where a minimum dose is required for effect. As they decrease the concentration, the medicine becomes less and less efficient. But below a threshold, the medicine starts getting potent again. Most homeopathic remedies may not even contain any pharmacologically active molecules anymore. Some describe it as an image or compare it to a fingerprint of the original medicine. Homeopathy can only be tracked by results. It helps to understand that if you were to test for hcg in your body by taking a pregnancy test, because you have not added actual hcg hormone to your body, it would not cause the test to conclude positive.

About the HCG Diet

The HCG diet, which is based on Dr. Simeons' "Pounds and Inches", has successfully aided in the weight loss of thousands for over 50 years. Previously, HCG was only available in an injection form which was administered at costly spas and medical weight loss clinics. It was only recently that homeopathic HCG became available in a sublingual form (no needles) giving everyday people an opportunity to experience this weight loss phenomenon. This diet is only done for a short period of time but achieves incredible results. Many people lose a pound a day. And if you have more to lose, you may do consecutive rounds of it again and again!

What you can expect from this diet plan

- Lose 20 to 40 pounds per month.
- Rapid, yet safe weight loss.
- No hunger.
- No exercise required.
- Simple easy to follow plan.
- Reprograms your brain to release stored fat.
- Resets your metabolism to normal.
- No unpleasant side effects.
- Learn how to maintain your desired weight.
- You will not be restricted to eating only certain foods for the rest of your life.

How HCG Drops Works

HCG diet drops are a sub-lingual homeopathic weight loss formula that is taken orally. Drops are placed under the tongue and are rapidly absorbed into your system. This triggers your body to subsist more on your stored fat rather than on what you eat. It causes the body to release the stored fat or "food" taken from the fat that is being broken down in your body. This allows the burning of 3500 to 4000 calories of fat stored in your body, which equates to the loss of 1 to 2 pounds in a day!

Instructions for use:

Look in a mirror and drop 10 individual little drops (don't squirt) into your mouth, under the tongue. Do this 30 minutes before each meal. Make sure to hold the drops under your tongue for 2- 5 minutes and don't drink anything or brush your teeth for 15 minutes before or after taking the drops. Do this three times a day.

How HCG Pellets Are Used

HCG Pellets are a sub-lingual homeopathic weight loss formula that **work the same way as the oral drops, but are a bit more convenient. Simply let 4 pellets dissolve under your tongue three times a day. This leads to more accurate dosing and skips the need for a mirror to administer the dose. Same rules apply, no drinks 15 minutes before or after taking the pellets!**

Preparation for the Diet

Before you get started on your HCG Diet Program, decide if you want to do a colon cleanse. If you have time, it will

certainly increase your results! But if you don't, don't worry!
Many pounds have been lost without prior cleansing!
Chose a start date. Any time when you have 3 weeks free
and clear from food focused events would be good. If you
are a woman, wait until after your menstrual cycle has finished for best results.

Shop for what you will need:

- Homeopathic Drops or Pellets
- Vitamin B12 (for energy)
- Potassium Supplement
- Non-oil based body products (no fat in or on your
  body)

HCG Phase 1
Load Days

I know it sounds "unreal"! But for the first two days of the diet, **you get to gorge on all the fatty foods you can force down your throat!** Focus on Fat! Not sugar! Eat as much as you can throughout the day. The more you eat and the higher the fat content, the better. Keep in mind that the purpose of this two day "gorge" is to better assist your body's fat reserve to open up and start releasing extra calories throughout Phase 2. as well as to keep you from getting hungry when your food intake is very limited!

Note: Do not try to skip this phase thinking you do not want to gain anymore weight! You will set yourself up for failure, because you will be hungry during the whole diet and you will eventually give in and quit! So don't do it! You will gain a few pounds for these two days, but it will come off fast in the next few days. I personally have tried it both ways and know this from experience!

During this gorge, make sure you start taking your HCG drops or pellets. You will want to spread out the dosage times throughout the day. Take ten drops or 4 pellets in the morning, then before lunch and again before dinner. I know you will be eating all day long, but pause long enough to allow for 30 minutes prior to eating, three times a day.

HCG Phase 2
VLCD - Very Low Calorie Diet

Here's the heart of the HCG Diet. Starting on the third day of using your drops or pellets, you will be reducing your food intake to 500 calories. Shocking, I know! But have no fear... as you are very well aware, you will not be hungry! **The HCG is already working in your body and though you tried to pig out yesterday, you just weren't that hungry!** So the switch to the VLCD is a breeze! Your brain will think you want more, but you stomach will be totally satisfied!

Note: It is very important to follow the HCG diet protocol to the tee or you will experience lower weight loss results! HCG by itself does not produce any weight loss results**! It simply stops your hunger allowing you to stay on a ridiculously low calorie diet.** As a bonus, it encourages your body to release stored, unwanted fat.

Follow the Diet protocol outlined below starting on day 3. Continue for three weeks (or until day 23). You may continue longer if you choose for up to 40 days on phase 2 (or until day 42).

Eat only from the foods listed here and don't skip any meals! Your total intake will be around 500 calorie consisting of protein, vegetables and fruits. Don't worry; **the HCG will make your body release an additional 1500 to 4000 calories from stored fat** so you will burn an acceptable amount of calories.

Important reminders for Phase 2:
- **Drink lots of water!** This is critical if you are going to flush that unwanted fat from your body. Your fat storehouses

will be releasing it, but you can help it exit your body! Aim to drink a ½ gallon or more of water a day. (Eight 8 ounce glasses a day).

- **Do not do any strenuous exercise while on Phase 2!** You may walk for 30 minutes daily. You are either going to love or hate this. To those of us who don't like to exercise, you may be thinking that you just died and went to heaven! Has anyone ever told you not to exercise?! I know! I know! This is very cool! If you are on the other side of the fence here, you may be saying, "What?! Change my whole routine?" I would just like to remind you, it is only for 3 weeks and isn't losing 20 pounds or more worth it? But if you must exercise, keep it light, very light! Some who just can't live without their exercise try to up their protein a little bit. But speaking from experience, doing exercise while on HCG can cause quite a bit of pain!
- **Do not use any cosmetics other than lipstick, eyebrow pencil and powder.** Remember, you don't want any fats and oils entering your body through your mouth or your skin because it will affect your weight loss. This includes lotions as well! There are HCG approved products available. You can pick them up at a local health supplement store or you can order them from www.myhcgsource.com.
- **Keep taking your prescribed medications.** Most people report having great results on the HCG Diet while continuing to take prescription medication. Be sure to have you blood work done by your doctor after you finish your diet because he may need to lower the dosage of your meds. Some of the benefits of this diet tend to be lower blood pressure and lower blood sugar levels!
- **Vitamins are permitted and it is recommended that you take Vitamin B-12 daily.** You will need this for energy.

Potassium is also recommended because it will help your cells to release fluids and it can assist you in your weight loss. Without it, you may get headaches and leg cramps.

- **Stay away from diet sodas.** I know they have zero calories, but that is not the problem. The artificial sweeteners will spike insulin levels and make your body hold on to fat. And we don't want that, do we?! Stevia is the recommended sweetener while on this diet.
- **If you lose more than 34 pounds** total during this period, stop phase 2 immediately and move on the phase 3.

NOTE: Though you will be eating small quantities of food, do not despair. You will find that you will be satisfied with these quantities. If you ask yourself, "How do I feel?" The answer will surprise you! You are just fine! You really are not hungry. As day turns to night, each meal will come with a surprise of the notion that you really are not that hungry! In the past, diets like this would scare the daylights out of you, and if you are just checking this out for the first time, you are probably thinking of closing this book and saying, "Forget it!" Don't give up until you try it! The HCG will truly help control your appetite! Don't underestimate it.

Breakfast: No food. Drink as much coffee and tea without sugar as you like. Only one tablespoon of milk allowed in 24 hours. Stevia may be used.

Lunch: Choose 1 Protein, 1 Vegetable, 1 Fruit and 1 Bread serving.

Dinner: Choose 1 Protein, 1 Vegetable, 1 Fruit and 1 Bread serving.

Choose one food from each of the four categories. No more than 4 foods can be eaten at any meal.

Protein	Vegetable
Choose only <u>one</u> protein for lunch and for dinner. Never eat the same protein twice on the same day. Weigh 100 grams prior to cooking. Beef, veal, chicken breast (no skin), shrimp, lobster, crab, whitefish (Flounder, Sole, Sea Bass, Orange Roughy, Tilapia, Halibut)	Choose only <u>one</u> vegetable for lunch and another for dinner. Never eat the same vegetable in the same day. Tomato, celery, lettuce, spinach, cucumbers, onions, cabbage, asparagus, chard, radishes, beet greens.
Fruit	**Bread**
Choose only <u>one</u> fruit for lunch and another for dinner. Never eat the same fruit twice on the same day. May be eaten between meals as a snack. ½ grapefruit, ½ cup strawberries, 1 medium orange, 1 medium apple.	Choose a bread for lunch and again for dinner. May be eaten between meals as a snack. 1 Melba Toast, 2 Melba Rounds, 1 Grissini or Alessi Breadstick.

Liquids – Drink as much coffee, tea, herb tea and water as you like throughout the day.

Seasonings – The juice of one lemon daily is allowed for all purposes. Vinegar, salt, pepper, mustard powder, garlic, sweet basil, parsley, thyme, marjoram, etc., may be used for seasoning. No oil, butter, or dressing. Stevia can be used to sweeten foods and is available in a variety of flavors.

HCG Phase 3
Maintenance

Phase 3 is, hands down, the most important phase of this diet! Even more so than the VLCD on Phase 2! Yes, you have lost a lot of weight and I'm sure you are ready to eat everything you have been denying yourself of, but hold up! Follow these instructions carefully! **You need to maintain your weight loss for 3 weeks.** Most people don't realize how vital this part is in resetting the hypothalamus gland. You do not want to gain or lose during this stage! **If the scale moves more than 2 pounds in either direction, you will not establish a new set point!** And all this effort will have been for nothing! What is a set point? It is the weight at which your body (not you), likes to hang around at! In the past, we may have dieted, lost weight, and gained it back again. **The trick to not gaining it back is to stay at the same weight for at least 3 weeks!** Do not miss this point! If you continue loosing weight, the new set point will never be set! If you go back to eating lots of carbs, fats, and sugars, the new set point will never be set!

Important reminders for Phase 3:

- Stop taking HCG
- Continue to stay on the 500 calorie diet for 3 days until the HCG has exited your body.
- After 3 days, you may increase your calorie intake to 1500 to 2000. You may start adding in eggs, cheese and healthy fats like olive oil.
- Do not eat any sugar or starches for 3 weeks.
- If you gain more than 2 pounds from the last weight you recorded while on HCG you must do a "steak day".

Steak Day
1 large apple at lunch.
6 ounces of steak and 1 tomato at dinner. * Steak day can be done anytime in phase 2 if you need to break a plateau.

HCG Phase 4
Healthy Lifestyle

Phase 4 is really in effect, what you do for the rest of your life. You need to take it easy here and slowly introduce healthy foods back into your diet. **Slowly start adding starches and sugar, in small quantities, to your diet.** The key to this is slowly! Be mindful to only eat small portions of carbohydrates. You don't want to balloon up again, right? Keep your eye on the scale, too, but your focus will be on optimal health. You will find that smaller amounts of food will satisfy you now. You will feel fuller, faster. Listen to you new sense of less hunger and do not eat when you are not hungry. Enjoy your new slender body!

How to use this book

As you start this diet, you will receive the simple advice you need daily to be successful. Each morning during the diet, you will want to weigh yourself. Simply record your weight in this log book and keep track of the foods you are eating. Keep track of your water intake as well. By keeping a log you will be sure to stay on track, eating the proper foods at the proper times. As each day dawns, you will be encouraged by seeing your weight loss results in front of your face daily! Every day will reward you with certain success!

Day 1

Today's Date_____

(Gorge Day!)

Starting Weight_____

Take your HCG Drops three times a day.
Eat! Go ahead; eat as much fatty food that your heart de-
sires! Then eat some more! Don't make yourself sick though.

We're not kidding here. Stuffing yourself to the gills is an essential part of this diet. It comes right at that start, *before* you start limiting yourself to 500 calories per day. On these first 2 days you'll stuff thousands of calories into your body. You'll start taking your hCG as directed, but you'll hardly notice it between all those fatty foods. That's what you're going for: calories that come from fat. You don't want a whole lot of sugar, but you can pack in the fat like crazy.

Gorging is the key to this diet. The hCG diet works because it takes your hunger away, and leaves you with a satisfying diet of 500 calories per day. But those calories will only satisfy you if you begin the process with a full-scale fat gorge. The hCG needs the fat to make the diet work. If you skip it, you will be hungry, and, as with most diets, you will be left with only your will power to fight off a ravenous appetite. You've already lost that battle plenty of times. That's why you're trying this new strategy. So get over it, and let yourself go. Eat burgers, fried foods, mashed potatoes—anything that's not high on sweets, but has plenty of fat. With a proper 2-day gorge, and the proper dosage of hCG you'll be on your way.

TIP of the DAY
During the gorge days, eat everything fatty that you have always wanted. Don't worry about gaining! It will come right back off, I promise!

Day 2

(Gorge Day!)

**Take your HCG drops 3 times a day.
Keep Eating! Fill that gut with as much fatty food as you can pack in it! Just don't make yourself sick!**

Are you finding it difficult to eat? You should! That HCG is revved up and working big time in your body! And it's only day 2! **Even if you don't feel hungry, still eat!** And make sure it's fatty food, not sugary foods. Today is your last chance to pig out and have all those yummy foods you know you should stay away from!

Breakfast: Go eat a cheesy omelet, hash browns, sausage, creamy latte, leftover pizza…! Anything goes, just make sure it is full of fat!

Don't wait for lunch… Go get a donut! Heck, go get a whole dozen and have a donut party with everyone that you are with!

Lunch time! Hmmm… What to eat? A big juicy burger, cheesy pizza, French fries, Nachos and cheese, loaded potato skins…

Snack time! Raid that vending machine!

Dinner time! Go to your favorite restaurant and get your best "last meal"!

Dessert! "Move on over dinner, because I need to throw down some cheesecake!" Your choice of dessert.

TIP of the DAY
Don't skip the gorge days! If you do, you will feel hungry during phase 2. If you are hungry, you will fall off the diet!

Day 3
(1ˢᵗ day of 500 calorie diet)

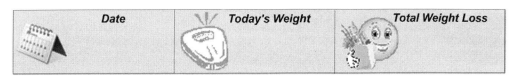

Date	Today's Weight	Total Weight Loss

Breakfast -- stay full drinking any amount of tea, coffee, or water.
(it all counts towards your total water for the day.)

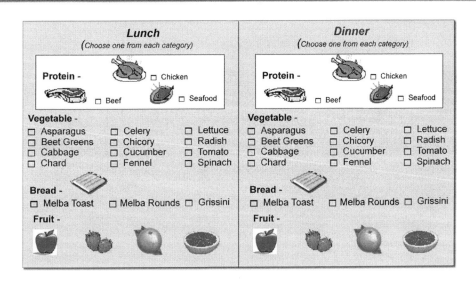

Lunch
(Choose one from each category)

Protein -
☐ Chicken
☐ Beef   ☐ Seafood

Vegetable -
☐ Asparagus   ☐ Celery   ☐ Lettuce
☐ Beet Greens   ☐ Chicory   ☐ Radish
☐ Cabbage   ☐ Cucumber   ☐ Tomato
☐ Chard   ☐ Fennel   ☐ Spinach

Bread -
☐ Melba Toast   ☐ Melba Rounds   ☐ Grissini

Fruit -

Dinner
(Choose one from each category)

Protein -
☐ Chicken
☐ Beef   ☐ Seafood

Vegetable -
☐ Asparagus   ☐ Celery   ☐ Lettuce
☐ Beet Greens   ☐ Chicory   ☐ Radish
☐ Cabbage   ☐ Cucumber   ☐ Tomato
☐ Chard   ☐ Fennel   ☐ Spinach

Bread -
☐ Melba Toast   ☐ Melba Rounds   ☐ Grissini

Fruit -

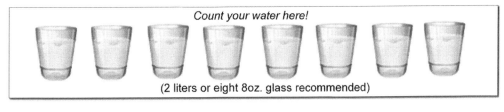

Count your water here!

(2 liters or eight 8oz. glass recommended)

Comments for Today _____

_____

_____

_____

_____

TIP of the DAY
Listen to your stomach! Your mind will say, "Yikes! I need to eat! This won't be enough!" But listen to your stomach. Just chill. Really, you're not really that hungry!

19

Day 4

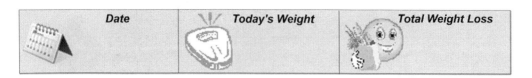

Date	Today's Weight	Total Weight Loss

Breakfast -- stay full drinking any amount of tea, coffee, or water.
(it all counts towards your total water for the day.)

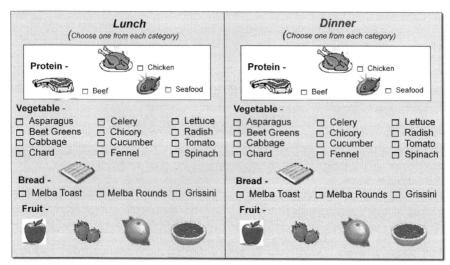

Lunch
(Choose one from each category)

Protein -
☐ Chicken
☐ Beef
☐ Seafood

Vegetable -
☐ Asparagus ☐ Celery ☐ Lettuce
☐ Beet Greens ☐ Chicory ☐ Radish
☐ Cabbage ☐ Cucumber ☐ Tomato
☐ Chard ☐ Fennel ☐ Spinach

Bread -
☐ Melba Toast ☐ Melba Rounds ☐ Grissini

Fruit -

Dinner
(Choose one from each category)

Protein -
☐ Chicken
☐ Beef
☐ Seafood

Vegetable -
☐ Asparagus ☐ Celery ☐ Lettuce
☐ Beet Greens ☐ Chicory ☐ Radish
☐ Cabbage ☐ Cucumber ☐ Tomato
☐ Chard ☐ Fennel ☐ Spinach

Bread -
☐ Melba Toast ☐ Melba Rounds ☐ Grissini

Fruit -

Count your water here!

(2 liters or eight 8oz. glass recommended)

Comments for Today

TIP of the DAY

Try to buy organic as recommended by HCG diet experts. But if you can't, for whatever reason, don't worry! Many people have had success on this diet without doing it that way.

Day 5

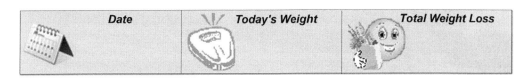

Date	Today's Weight	Total Weight Loss

Breakfast -- stay full drinking any amount of tea, coffee, or water.
(it all counts towards your total water for the day.)

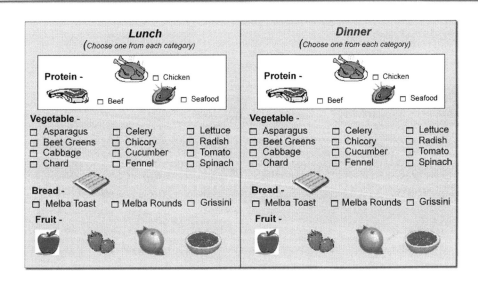

Lunch
(Choose one from each category)

Protein -
☐ Chicken
☐ Beef
☐ Seafood

Vegetable -
☐ Asparagus   ☐ Celery   ☐ Lettuce
☐ Beet Greens   ☐ Chicory   ☐ Radish
☐ Cabbage   ☐ Cucumber   ☐ Tomato
☐ Chard   ☐ Fennel   ☐ Spinach

Bread -
☐ Melba Toast   ☐ Melba Rounds   ☐ Grissini

Fruit -

Dinner
(Choose one from each category)

Protein -
☐ Chicken
☐ Beef
☐ Seafood

Vegetable -
☐ Asparagus   ☐ Celery   ☐ Lettuce
☐ Beet Greens   ☐ Chicory   ☐ Radish
☐ Cabbage   ☐ Cucumber   ☐ Tomato
☐ Chard   ☐ Fennel   ☐ Spinach

Bread -
☐ Melba Toast   ☐ Melba Rounds   ☐ Grissini

Fruit -

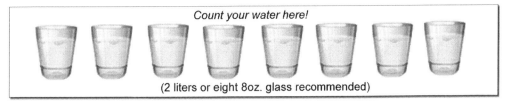

Count your water here!

(2 liters or eight 8oz. glass recommended)

Comments for Today

TIP of the DAY
Don't bore your taste buds! You're only eating small portions so make it taste good! Get some great tasting recipes from my book, "Easy, Breezy Weight Loss on the HCG Diet" or check out my video recipe blog at www.myhcgsource.com.

Day 7

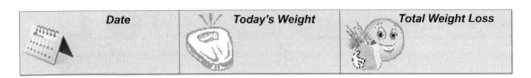

Date	Today's Weight	Total Weight Loss

Breakfast -- stay full drinking any amount of tea, coffee, or water.
(it all counts towards your total water for the day.)

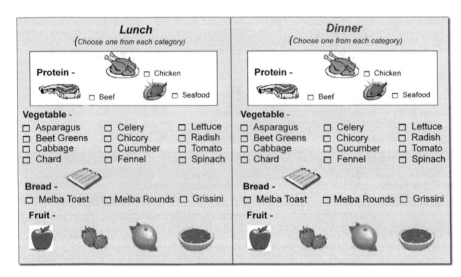

Lunch
(Choose one from each category)

Protein -
☐ Chicken
☐ Beef
☐ Seafood

Vegetable -
☐ Asparagus ☐ Celery ☐ Lettuce
☐ Beet Greens ☐ Chicory ☐ Radish
☐ Cabbage ☐ Cucumber ☐ Tomato
☐ Chard ☐ Fennel ☐ Spinach

Bread -
☐ Melba Toast ☐ Melba Rounds ☐ Grissini

Fruit -

Dinner
(Choose one from each category)

Protein -
☐ Chicken
☐ Beef
☐ Seafood

Vegetable -
☐ Asparagus ☐ Celery ☐ Lettuce
☐ Beet Greens ☐ Chicory ☐ Radish
☐ Cabbage ☐ Cucumber ☐ Tomato
☐ Chard ☐ Fennel ☐ Spinach

Bread -
☐ Melba Toast ☐ Melba Rounds ☐ Grissini

Fruit -

Count your water here!

(2 liters or eight 8oz. glass recommended)

Comments for Today

TIP of the DAY

Make sure you change up your food selection at every meal. If you have chicken at lunch, choose beef or fish at dinner. If you have tomatoes at lunch, choose something else, like spinach, at dinner.

Day 8

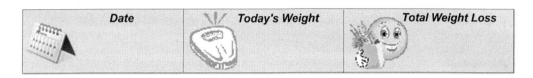

	Date		Today's Weight		Total Weight Loss

Breakfast -- stay full drinking any amount of tea, coffee, or water.
(it all counts towards your total water for the day.)

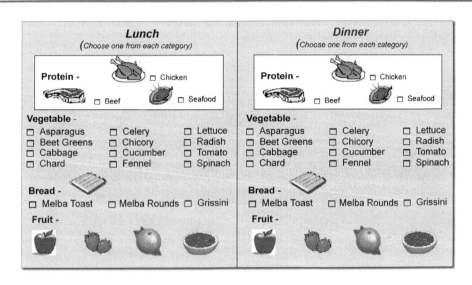

Lunch
(Choose one from each category)

Protein -
☐ Chicken
☐ Beef   ☐ Seafood

Vegetable -
☐ Asparagus   ☐ Celery   ☐ Lettuce
☐ Beet Greens   ☐ Chicory   ☐ Radish
☐ Cabbage   ☐ Cucumber   ☐ Tomato
☐ Chard   ☐ Fennel   ☐ Spinach

Bread -
☐ Melba Toast   ☐ Melba Rounds   ☐ Grissini

Fruit -

Dinner
(Choose one from each category)

Protein -
☐ Chicken
☐ Beef   ☐ Seafood

Vegetable -
☐ Asparagus   ☐ Celery   ☐ Lettuce
☐ Beet Greens   ☐ Chicory   ☐ Radish
☐ Cabbage   ☐ Cucumber   ☐ Tomato
☐ Chard   ☐ Fennel   ☐ Spinach

Bread -
☐ Melba Toast   ☐ Melba Rounds   ☐ Grissini

Fruit -

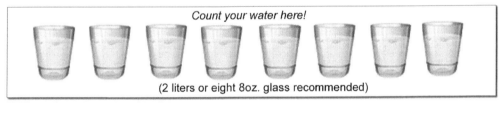

Count your water here!

(2 liters or eight 8oz. glass recommended)

Comments for Today

TIP of the DAY

If you are tempted to exercise, wait until you are on Phase 3 Maintenance. Nothing more than brisk walking is recommended when you are on Phase 2.

Day 9

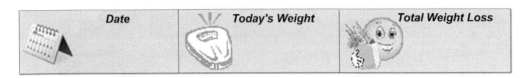

Date	Today's Weight	Total Weight Loss

Breakfast -- stay full drinking any amount of tea, coffee, or water.
(it all counts towards your total water for the day.)

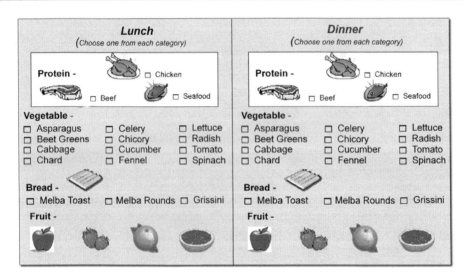

Lunch
(Choose one from each category)

Protein -
☐ Chicken
☐ Beef ☐ Seafood

Vegetable -
☐ Asparagus ☐ Celery ☐ Lettuce
☐ Beet Greens ☐ Chicory ☐ Radish
☐ Cabbage ☐ Cucumber ☐ Tomato
☐ Chard ☐ Fennel ☐ Spinach

Bread -
☐ Melba Toast ☐ Melba Rounds ☐ Grissini

Fruit -

Dinner
(Choose one from each category)

Protein -
☐ Chicken
☐ Beef ☐ Seafood

Vegetable -
☐ Asparagus ☐ Celery ☐ Lettuce
☐ Beet Greens ☐ Chicory ☐ Radish
☐ Cabbage ☐ Cucumber ☐ Tomato
☐ Chard ☐ Fennel ☐ Spinach

Bread -
☐ Melba Toast ☐ Melba Rounds ☐ Grissini

Fruit -

Count your water here!

(2 liters or eight 8oz. glass recommended)

Comments for Today

TIP of the DAY

Make sure you eat at regular intervals. If you wait too long to eat, you will probably feel hunger and are more likely to cheat.

Day 10

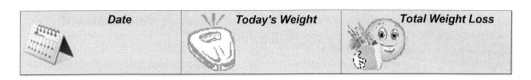

Date	Today's Weight	Total Weight Loss

Breakfast -- stay full drinking any amount of tea, coffee, or water.
(it all counts towards your total water for the day.)

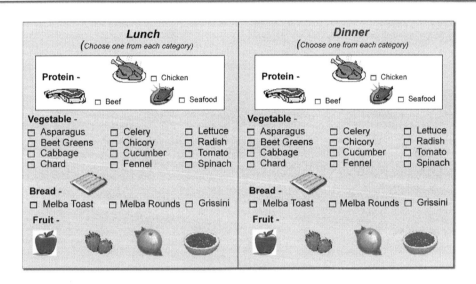

Lunch
(Choose one from each category)

Protein -
☐ Chicken
☐ Beef ☐ Seafood

Vegetable -
☐ Asparagus ☐ Celery ☐ Lettuce
☐ Beet Greens ☐ Chicory ☐ Radish
☐ Cabbage ☐ Cucumber ☐ Tomato
☐ Chard ☐ Fennel ☐ Spinach

Bread -
☐ Melba Toast ☐ Melba Rounds ☐ Grissini

Fruit -

Dinner
(Choose one from each category)

Protein -
☐ Chicken
☐ Beef ☐ Seafood

Vegetable -
☐ Asparagus ☐ Celery ☐ Lettuce
☐ Beet Greens ☐ Chicory ☐ Radish
☐ Cabbage ☐ Cucumber ☐ Tomato
☐ Chard ☐ Fennel ☐ Spinach

Bread -
☐ Melba Toast ☐ Melba Rounds ☐ Grissini

Fruit -

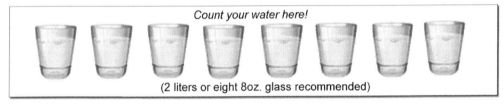

Count your water here!

(2 liters or eight 8oz. glass recommended)

Comments for Today

TIP of the DAY
Weigh yourself daily! The scale will be your cheerleader! On this diet, you should see an average of 1 to 2 pounds lost per day!

Day 11

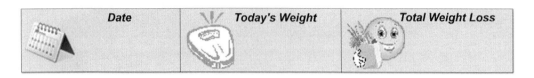

	Date		Today's Weight		Total Weight Loss

Breakfast -- stay full drinking any amount of tea, coffee, or water.
(it all counts towards your total water for the day.)

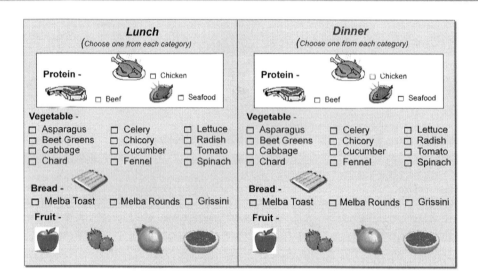

Lunch
(Choose one from each category)

Protein -
☐ Chicken
☐ Beef   ☐ Seafood

Vegetable -
☐ Asparagus   ☐ Celery   ☐ Lettuce
☐ Beet Greens   ☐ Chicory   ☐ Radish
☐ Cabbage   ☐ Cucumber   ☐ Tomato
☐ Chard   ☐ Fennel   ☐ Spinach

Bread -
☐ Melba Toast   ☐ Melba Rounds ☐ Grissini

Fruit -

Dinner
(Choose one from each category)

Protein -
☐ Chicken
☐ Beef   ☐ Seafood

Vegetable -
☐ Asparagus   ☐ Celery   ☐ Lettuce
☐ Beet Greens   ☐ Chicory   ☐ Radish
☐ Cabbage   ☐ Cucumber   ☐ Tomato
☐ Chard   ☐ Fennel   ☐ Spinach

Bread -
☐ Melba Toast   ☐ Melba Rounds ☐ Grissini

Fruit -

Count your water here!

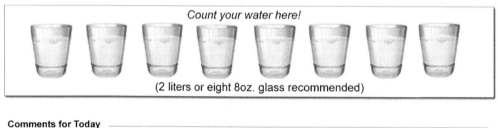

(2 liters or eight 8oz. glass recommended)

Comments for Today

TIP of the DAY

Don't cheat, like you may have done on other diets! There is a science to this diet and the slightest cheat will mess it up! It's not about the calories; it's about your body's switch to burning fat. Don't mess up the process!

Day 12

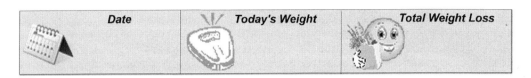

Date	Today's Weight	Total Weight Loss

Breakfast -- stay full drinking any amount of tea, coffee, or water.
(it all counts towards your total water for the day.)

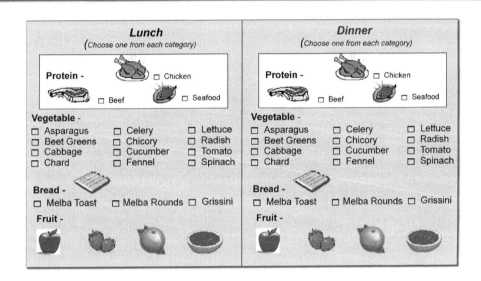

Lunch
(Choose one from each category)

Protein -
☐ Chicken
☐ Beef ☐ Seafood

Vegetable -
☐ Asparagus ☐ Celery ☐ Lettuce
☐ Beet Greens ☐ Chicory ☐ Radish
☐ Cabbage ☐ Cucumber ☐ Tomato
☐ Chard ☐ Fennel ☐ Spinach

Bread -
☐ Melba Toast ☐ Melba Rounds ☐ Grissini

Fruit -

Dinner
(Choose one from each category)

Protein -
☐ Chicken
☐ Beef ☐ Seafood

Vegetable -
☐ Asparagus ☐ Celery ☐ Lettuce
☐ Beet Greens ☐ Chicory ☐ Radish
☐ Cabbage ☐ Cucumber ☐ Tomato
☐ Chard ☐ Fennel ☐ Spinach

Bread -
☐ Melba Toast ☐ Melba Rounds ☐ Grissini

Fruit -

Count your water here!

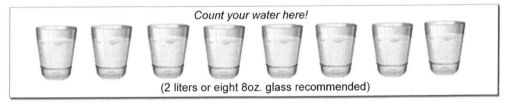

(2 liters or eight 8oz. glass recommended)

Comments for Today _____

_____

_____

_____

_____

TIP of the DAY

Don't use lotion or makeup while on Phase 2. No oils in your mouth or on your skin! The gorge kick started the fat burning process. You are now trying to starve it of fat so that it will burn your stored fat!

Day 13

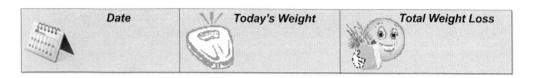

	Date		Today's Weight		Total Weight Loss

Breakfast -- stay full drinking any amount of tea, coffee, or water.
(it all counts towards your total water for the day.)

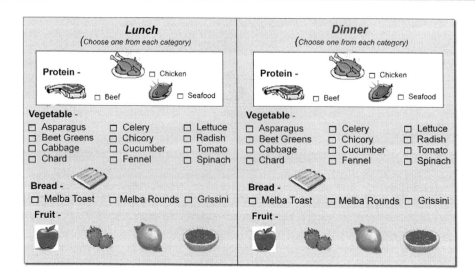

Lunch
(Choose one from each category)

Protein -
- ☐ Chicken
- ☐ Beef
- ☐ Seafood

Vegetable -
- ☐ Asparagus
- ☐ Beet Greens
- ☐ Cabbage
- ☐ Chard
- ☐ Celery
- ☐ Chicory
- ☐ Cucumber
- ☐ Fennel
- ☐ Lettuce
- ☐ Radish
- ☐ Tomato
- ☐ Spinach

Bread -
- ☐ Melba Toast
- ☐ Melba Rounds
- ☐ Grissini

Fruit -

Dinner
(Choose one from each category)

Protein -
- ☐ Chicken
- ☐ Beef
- ☐ Seafood

Vegetable -
- ☐ Asparagus
- ☐ Beet Greens
- ☐ Cabbage
- ☐ Chard
- ☐ Celery
- ☐ Chicory
- ☐ Cucumber
- ☐ Fennel
- ☐ Lettuce
- ☐ Radish
- ☐ Tomato
- ☐ Spinach

Bread -
- ☐ Melba Toast
- ☐ Melba Rounds
- ☐ Grissini

Fruit -

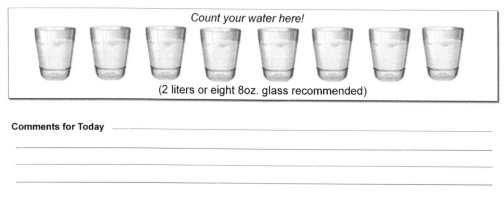

Count your water here!

(2 liters or eight 8oz. glass recommended)

Comments for Today

TIP of the DAY

When cooking, try sautéing your food in chicken broth or beef broth instead of oil or spray oil. It does the trick without the fat!

Day 14

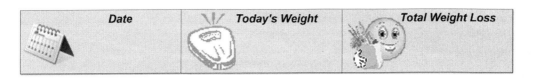

Date	Today's Weight	Total Weight Loss

Breakfast -- stay full drinking any amount of tea, coffee, or water.
(it all counts towards your total water for the day.)

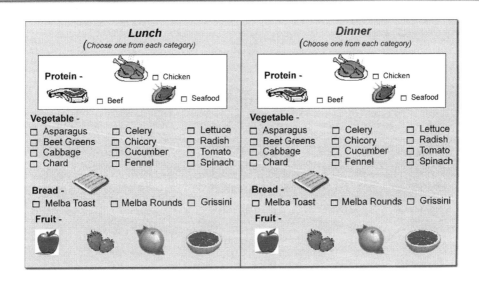

Lunch
(Choose one from each category)

Protein -
☐ Chicken
☐ Beef
☐ Seafood

Vegetable -
☐ Asparagus ☐ Celery ☐ Lettuce
☐ Beet Greens ☐ Chicory ☐ Radish
☐ Cabbage ☐ Cucumber ☐ Tomato
☐ Chard ☐ Fennel ☐ Spinach

Bread -
☐ Melba Toast ☐ Melba Rounds ☐ Grissini

Fruit -

Dinner
(Choose one from each category)

Protein -
☐ Chicken
☐ Beef
☐ Seafood

Vegetable -
☐ Asparagus ☐ Celery ☐ Lettuce
☐ Beet Greens ☐ Chicory ☐ Radish
☐ Cabbage ☐ Cucumber ☐ Tomato
☐ Chard ☐ Fennel ☐ Spinach

Bread -
☐ Melba Toast ☐ Melba Rounds ☐ Grissini

Fruit -

Count your water here!

(2 liters or eight 8oz. glass recommended)

Comments for Today _____

TIP of the DAY
Drink lots of fluids! You need to flush that fat out!

Day 15

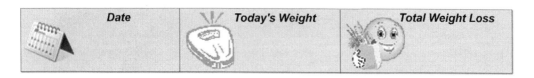

Date	Today's Weight	Total Weight Loss

Breakfast -- stay full drinking any amount of tea, coffee, or water.
(it all counts towards your total water for the day.)

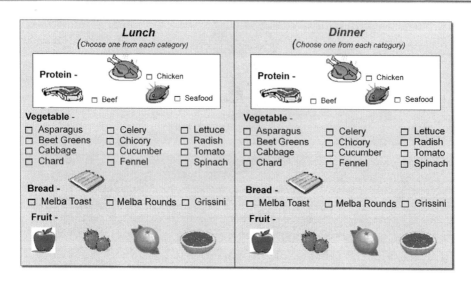

Lunch
(Choose one from each category)

Protein -
- ☐ Chicken
- ☐ Beef
- ☐ Seafood

Vegetable -
- ☐ Asparagus
- ☐ Beet Greens
- ☐ Cabbage
- ☐ Chard
- ☐ Celery
- ☐ Chicory
- ☐ Cucumber
- ☐ Fennel
- ☐ Lettuce
- ☐ Radish
- ☐ Tomato
- ☐ Spinach

Bread -
- ☐ Melba Toast
- ☐ Melba Rounds
- ☐ Grissini

Fruit -

Dinner
(Choose one from each category)

Protein -
- ☐ Chicken
- ☐ Beef
- ☐ Seafood

Vegetable -
- ☐ Asparagus
- ☐ Beet Greens
- ☐ Cabbage
- ☐ Chard
- ☐ Celery
- ☐ Chicory
- ☐ Cucumber
- ☐ Fennel
- ☐ Lettuce
- ☐ Radish
- ☐ Tomato
- ☐ Spinach

Bread -
- ☐ Melba Toast
- ☐ Melba Rounds
- ☐ Grissini

Fruit -

Count your water here!

(2 liters or eight 8oz. glass recommended)

Comments for Today

TIP of the DAY
Tell the waiter to have them prepare your food with no additional oils. They are usually happy to oblige.

Day 16

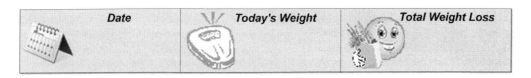

Date	Today's Weight	Total Weight Loss

Breakfast -- stay full drinking any amount of tea, coffee, or water.
(it all counts towards your total water for the day.)

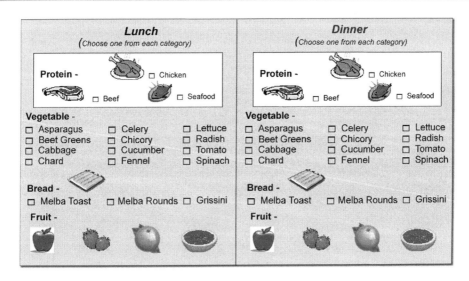

Lunch
(Choose one from each category)

Protein -
☐ Chicken
☐ Beef
☐ Seafood

Vegetable -
☐ Asparagus ☐ Celery ☐ Lettuce
☐ Beet Greens ☐ Chicory ☐ Radish
☐ Cabbage ☐ Cucumber ☐ Tomato
☐ Chard ☐ Fennel ☐ Spinach

Bread -
☐ Melba Toast ☐ Melba Rounds ☐ Grissini

Fruit -

Dinner
(Choose one from each category)

Protein -
☐ Chicken
☐ Beef
☐ Seafood

Vegetable -
☐ Asparagus ☐ Celery ☐ Lettuce
☐ Beet Greens ☐ Chicory ☐ Radish
☐ Cabbage ☐ Cucumber ☐ Tomato
☐ Chard ☐ Fennel ☐ Spinach

Bread -
☐ Melba Toast ☐ Melba Rounds ☐ Grissini

Fruit -

Count your water here!

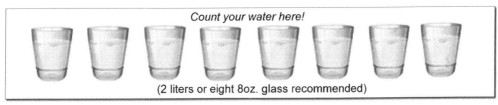

(2 liters or eight 8oz. glass recommended)

Comments for Today _____

TIP of the DAY
Skip the party if you can! Even though you are not hungry, the temptation is immense! But if you have to go, bring shrimp cocktail with lemon wedges on the side. You will need something "HCG Friendly" that you can eat as well.

Day 17

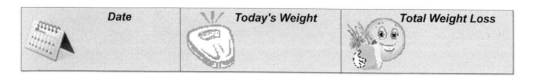

Date	Today's Weight	Total Weight Loss

Breakfast -- stay full drinking any amount of tea, coffee, or water.
(it all counts towards your total water for the day.)

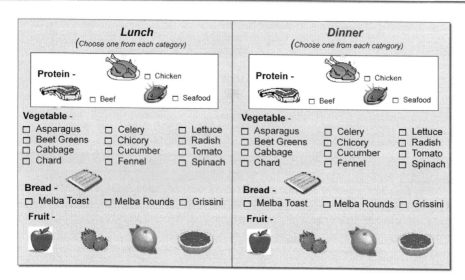

Lunch
(Choose one from each category)

Protein -
☐ Chicken
☐ Beef
☐ Seafood

Vegetable -
☐ Asparagus   ☐ Celery   ☐ Lettuce
☐ Beet Greens   ☐ Chicory   ☐ Radish
☐ Cabbage   ☐ Cucumber   ☐ Tomato
☐ Chard   ☐ Fennel   ☐ Spinach

Bread -
☐ Melba Toast   ☐ Melba Rounds   ☐ Grissini

Fruit -

Dinner
(Choose one from each category)

Protein -
☐ Chicken
☐ Beef
☐ Seafood

Vegetable -
☐ Asparagus   ☐ Celery   ☐ Lettuce
☐ Beet Greens   ☐ Chicory   ☐ Radish
☐ Cabbage   ☐ Cucumber   ☐ Tomato
☐ Chard   ☐ Fennel   ☐ Spinach

Bread -
☐ Melba Toast   ☐ Melba Rounds   ☐ Grissini

Fruit -

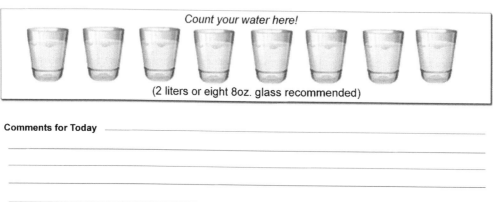

Count your water here!

(2 liters or eight 8oz. glass recommended)

Comments for Today

TIP of the DAY
Have emergency food ready in your fridge for when
you have no time to cook. Cut up celery or cucumbers.
Cooked chicken breast or pre packaged tuna.

Day 18

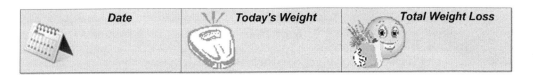

Date	Today's Weight	Total Weight Loss

Breakfast -- stay full drinking any amount of tea, coffee, or water.
(it all counts towards your total water for the day.)

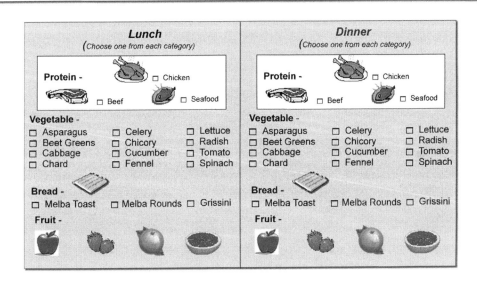

Lunch
(Choose one from each category)

Protein -
☐ Chicken
☐ Beef ☐ Seafood

Vegetable -
☐ Asparagus ☐ Celery ☐ Lettuce
☐ Beet Greens ☐ Chicory ☐ Radish
☐ Cabbage ☐ Cucumber ☐ Tomato
☐ Chard ☐ Fennel ☐ Spinach

Bread -
☐ Melba Toast ☐ Melba Rounds ☐ Grissini

Fruit -

Dinner
(Choose one from each category)

Protein -
☐ Chicken
☐ Beef ☐ Seafood

Vegetable -
☐ Asparagus ☐ Celery ☐ Lettuce
☐ Beet Greens ☐ Chicory ☐ Radish
☐ Cabbage ☐ Cucumber ☐ Tomato
☐ Chard ☐ Fennel ☐ Spinach

Bread -
☐ Melba Toast ☐ Melba Rounds ☐ Grissini

Fruit -

Count your water here!

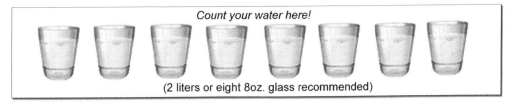

(2 liters or eight 8oz. glass recommended)

Comments for Today _____

_____

_____

_____

_____

_____

TIP of the DAY

Get flavored liquid stevia! It is so good! Add hazelnut stevia to coffee. Lemon drop stevia to water. Vanilla cream to fruit smoothies. Yum! Available at www.myhcgsource.com.

Day 19

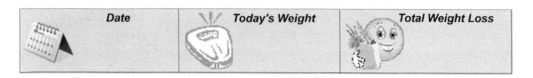

Date	Today's Weight	Total Weight Loss

Breakfast -- stay full drinking any amount of tea, coffee, or water.
(it all counts towards your total water for the day.)

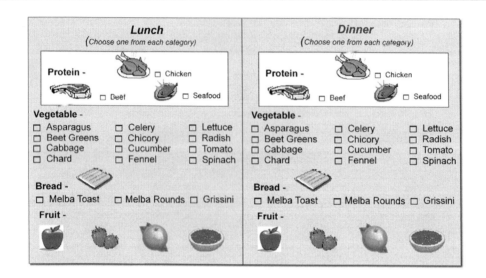

Lunch
(Choose one from each category)

Protein -
- ☐ Chicken
- ☐ Beef
- ☐ Seafood

Vegetable -
- ☐ Asparagus
- ☐ Beet Greens
- ☐ Cabbage
- ☐ Chard
- ☐ Celery
- ☐ Chicory
- ☐ Cucumber
- ☐ Fennel
- ☐ Lettuce
- ☐ Radish
- ☐ Tomato
- ☐ Spinach

Bread -
- ☐ Melba Toast   ☐ Melba Rounds   ☐ Grissini

Fruit -

Dinner
(Choose one from each category)

Protein -
- ☐ Chicken
- ☐ Beef
- ☐ Seafood

Vegetable -
- ☐ Asparagus
- ☐ Beet Greens
- ☐ Cabbage
- ☐ Chard
- ☐ Celery
- ☐ Chicory
- ☐ Cucumber
- ☐ Fennel
- ☐ Lettuce
- ☐ Radish
- ☐ Tomato
- ☐ Spinach

Bread -
- ☐ Melba Toast   ☐ Melba Rounds   ☐ Grissini

Fruit -

Count your water here!

(2 liters or eight 8oz. glass recommended)

Comments for Today

TIP of the DAY

Eat your fruit and bread between meals. You will find your stomach will be satisfied with the small portion at mealtime and it's something to look forward to in a few hours!

Day 20

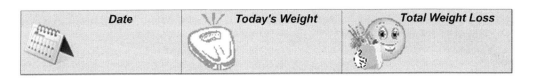

Date	Today's Weight	Total Weight Loss

Breakfast -- stay full drinking any amount of tea, coffee, or water.
(it all counts towards your total water for the day.)

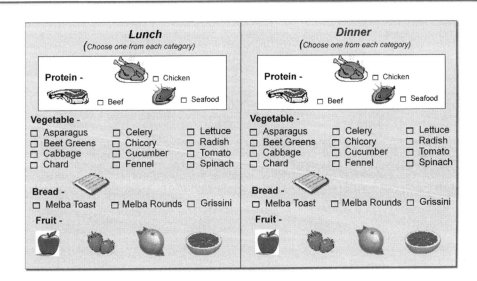

Lunch
(Choose one from each category)

Protein -
☐ Chicken
☐ Beef
☐ Seafood

Vegetable -
☐ Asparagus   ☐ Celery   ☐ Lettuce
☐ Beet Greens   ☐ Chicory   ☐ Radish
☐ Cabbage   ☐ Cucumber   ☐ Tomato
☐ Chard   ☐ Fennel   ☐ Spinach

Bread -
☐ Melba Toast   ☐ Melba Rounds   ☐ Grissini

Fruit -

Dinner
(Choose one from each category)

Protein -
☐ Chicken
☐ Beef
☐ Seafood

Vegetable -
☐ Asparagus   ☐ Celery   ☐ Lettuce
☐ Beet Greens   ☐ Chicory   ☐ Radish
☐ Cabbage   ☐ Cucumber   ☐ Tomato
☐ Chard   ☐ Fennel   ☐ Spinach

Bread -
☐ Melba Toast   ☐ Melba Rounds   ☐ Grissini

Fruit -

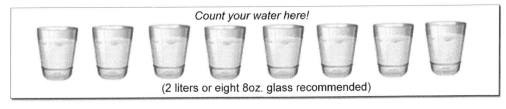

Count your water here!

(2 liters or eight 8oz. glass recommended)

Comments for Today

TIP of the DAY
Frozen shrimp cocktail is thawed out by lunchtime and feels like an elegant lunch!

Day 21

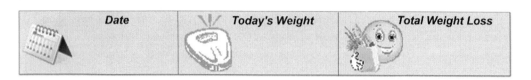

Date	Today's Weight	Total Weight Loss

Breakfast -- stay full drinking any amount of tea, coffee, or water.
(it all counts towards your total water for the day.)

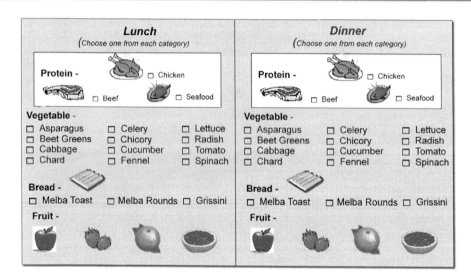

Lunch
(Choose one from each category)

Protein -
☐ Chicken
☐ Beef   ☐ Seafood

Vegetable -
☐ Asparagus   ☐ Celery   ☐ Lettuce
☐ Beet Greens   ☐ Chicory   ☐ Radish
☐ Cabbage   ☐ Cucumber   ☐ Tomato
☐ Chard   ☐ Fennel   ☐ Spinach

Bread -
☐ Melba Toast   ☐ Melba Rounds ☐ Grissini

Fruit -

Dinner
(Choose one from each category)

Protein -
☐ Chicken
☐ Beef   ☐ Seafood

Vegetable -
☐ Asparagus   ☐ Celery   ☐ Lettuce
☐ Beet Greens   ☐ Chicory   ☐ Radish
☐ Cabbage   ☐ Cucumber   ☐ Tomato
☐ Chard   ☐ Fennel   ☐ Spinach

Bread -
☐ Melba Toast   ☐ Melba Rounds ☐ Grissini

Fruit -

Count your water here!

(2 liters or eight 8oz. glass recommended)

Comments for Today

TIP of the DAY
Sea Salt is more flavorful than regular salt! Try it while you are on this diet, you will savor every bite!

Day 22

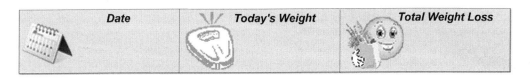

Date	Today's Weight	Total Weight Loss

Breakfast -- stay full drinking any amount of tea, coffee, or water.
(it all counts towards your total water for the day.)

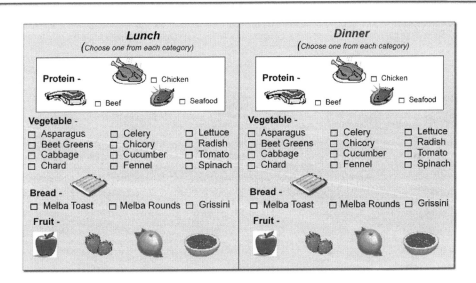

Lunch
(Choose one from each category)

Protein -
☐ Chicken
☐ Beef   ☐ Seafood

Vegetable -
☐ Asparagus   ☐ Celery   ☐ Lettuce
☐ Beet Greens ☐ Chicory   ☐ Radish
☐ Cabbage   ☐ Cucumber ☐ Tomato
☐ Chard   ☐ Fennel   ☐ Spinach

Bread -
☐ Melba Toast   ☐ Melba Rounds ☐ Grissini

Fruit -

Dinner
(Choose one from each category)

Protein -
☐ Chicken
☐ Beef   ☐ Seafood

Vegetable -
☐ Asparagus   ☐ Celery   ☐ Lettuce
☐ Beet Greens ☐ Chicory   ☐ Radish
☐ Cabbage   ☐ Cucumber ☐ Tomato
☐ Chard   ☐ Fennel   ☐ Spinach

Bread -
☐ Melba Toast   ☐ Melba Rounds ☐ Grissini

Fruit -

Count your water here!

(2 liters or eight 8oz. glass recommended)

Comments for Today

TIP of the DAY

Make sure you are taking a B-12 supplement while on this very low calorie diet! You are not getting enough in your diet and you will need the energy from it.

Day 23

(21ˢᵗ day of Phase 2 – 500 calorie diet)

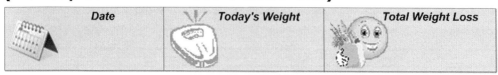

Date	Today's Weight	Total Weight Loss

Breakfast -- stay full drinking any amount of tea, coffee, or water.
(it all counts towards your total water for the day.)

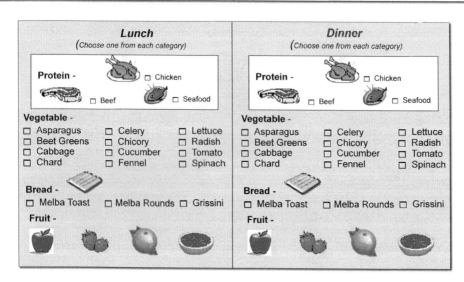

Lunch
(Choose one from each category)

Protein -
☐ Chicken
☐ Beef
☐ Seafood

Vegetable -
☐ Asparagus ☐ Celery ☐ Lettuce
☐ Beet Greens ☐ Chicory ☐ Radish
☐ Cabbage ☐ Cucumber ☐ Tomato
☐ Chard ☐ Fennel ☐ Spinach

Bread -
☐ Melba Toast ☐ Melba Rounds ☐ Grissini

Fruit -

Dinner
(Choose one from each category)

Protein -
☐ Chicken
☐ Beef
☐ Seafood

Vegetable -
☐ Asparagus ☐ Celery ☐ Lettuce
☐ Beet Greens ☐ Chicory ☐ Radish
☐ Cabbage ☐ Cucumber ☐ Tomato
☐ Chard ☐ Fennel ☐ Spinach

Bread -
☐ Melba Toast ☐ Melba Rounds ☐ Grissini

Fruit -

Count your water here!

(2 liters or eight 8oz. glass recommended)

Comments for Today

TIP of the DAY

Anytime after day 23 you can stop Phase 2. Follow instructions for day 41, 42 and 43. Then skip ahead to Phase 3 Maintenance. If you wish, you may continue on the 500 calorie diet until day 43.

Day 24

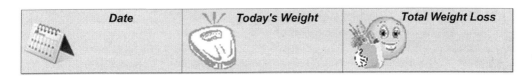

Date	Today's Weight	Total Weight Loss

Breakfast -- stay full drinking any amount of tea, coffee, or water.
(it all counts towards your total water for the day.)

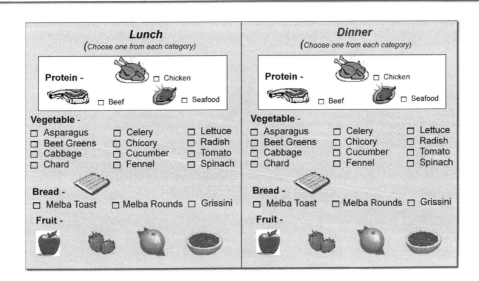

Lunch
(Choose one from each category)

Protein -
- ☐ Chicken
- ☐ Beef
- ☐ Seafood

Vegetable -
- ☐ Asparagus
- ☐ Beet Greens
- ☐ Cabbage
- ☐ Chard
- ☐ Celery
- ☐ Chicory
- ☐ Cucumber
- ☐ Fennel
- ☐ Lettuce
- ☐ Radish
- ☐ Tomato
- ☐ Spinach

Bread -
- ☐ Melba Toast
- ☐ Melba Rounds
- ☐ Grissini

Fruit -

Dinner
(Choose one from each category)

Protein -
- ☐ Chicken
- ☐ Beef
- ☐ Seafood

Vegetable -
- ☐ Asparagus
- ☐ Beet Greens
- ☐ Cabbage
- ☐ Chard
- ☐ Celery
- ☐ Chicory
- ☐ Cucumber
- ☐ Fennel
- ☐ Lettuce
- ☐ Radish
- ☐ Tomato
- ☐ Spinach

Bread -
- ☐ Melba Toast
- ☐ Melba Rounds
- ☐ Grissini

Fruit -

Count your water here!

(2 liters or eight 8oz. glass recommended)

Comments for Today

TIP of the DAY

Be ready to combat the "diet hecklers". Yes, you could lose weight on a 500 calorie diet without the HCG, but no one could ever last on it, because without the HCG, you would be so hungry that you would eventually give out and quit the diet!

Day 25

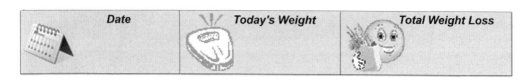

Date	Today's Weight	Total Weight Loss

Breakfast -- stay full drinking any amount of tea, coffee, or water.
(it all counts towards your total water for the day.)

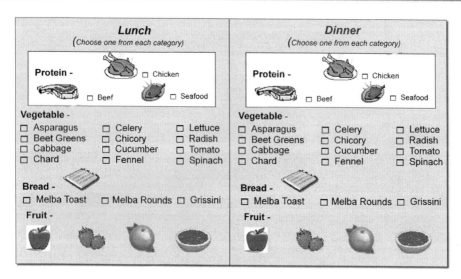

Lunch
(Choose one from each category)

Protein -
☐ Chicken
☐ Beef
☐ Seafood

Vegetable -
☐ Asparagus ☐ Celery ☐ Lettuce
☐ Beet Greens ☐ Chicory ☐ Radish
☐ Cabbage ☐ Cucumber ☐ Tomato
☐ Chard ☐ Fennel ☐ Spinach

Bread -
☐ Melba Toast ☐ Melba Rounds ☐ Grissini

Fruit -

Dinner
(Choose one from each category)

Protein -
☐ Chicken
☐ Beef
☐ Seafood

Vegetable -
☐ Asparagus ☐ Celery ☐ Lettuce
☐ Beet Greens ☐ Chicory ☐ Radish
☐ Cabbage ☐ Cucumber ☐ Tomato
☐ Chard ☐ Fennel ☐ Spinach

Bread -
☐ Melba Toast ☐ Melba Rounds ☐ Grissini

Fruit -

Count your water here!

(2 liters or eight 8oz. glass recommended)

Comments for Today

TIP of the DAY

It is believed that homeopathic HCG is a safe alternative to the actual HCG hormone which is only available with a prescription. Homeopathic HCG provides the same great results, but it will not show up on a pregnancy test.

Day 26

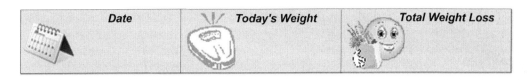

Date	Today's Weight	Total Weight Loss

Breakfast -- stay full drinking any amount of tea, coffee, or water.
(it all counts towards your total water for the day.)

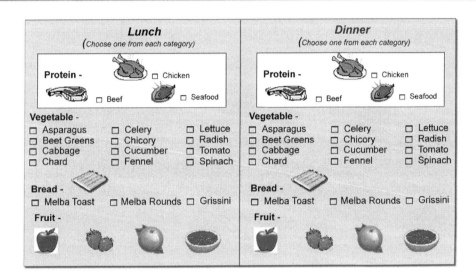

Lunch
(Choose one from each category)

Protein -
☐ Chicken
☐ Beef
☐ Seafood

Vegetable -
☐ Asparagus ☐ Celery ☐ Lettuce
☐ Beet Greens ☐ Chicory ☐ Radish
☐ Cabbage ☐ Cucumber ☐ Tomato
☐ Chard ☐ Fennel ☐ Spinach

Bread -
☐ Melba Toast ☐ Melba Rounds ☐ Grissini

Fruit -

Dinner
(Choose one from each category)

Protein -
☐ Chicken
☐ Beef
☐ Seafood

Vegetable -
☐ Asparagus ☐ Celery ☐ Lettuce
☐ Beet Greens ☐ Chicory ☐ Radish
☐ Cabbage ☐ Cucumber ☐ Tomato
☐ Chard ☐ Fennel ☐ Spinach

Bread -
☐ Melba Toast ☐ Melba Rounds ☐ Grissini

Fruit -

Count your water here!

(2 liters or eight 8oz. glass recommended)

Comments for Today

TIP of the DAY
If you snack late-night under normal conditions, and you are having a tough time with that while on this diet, try going to bed earlier. You've been wanting to catch up on some good sleep anyways!

Day 27

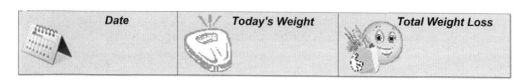

Date	Today's Weight	Total Weight Loss

Breakfast -- stay full drinking any amount of tea, coffee, or water.
(it all counts towards your total water for the day.)

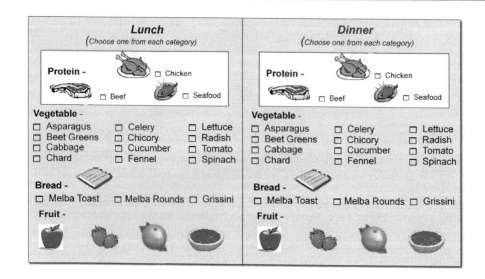

Lunch
(Choose one from each category)

Protein -
☐ Chicken
☐ Beef ☐ Seafood

Vegetable -
☐ Asparagus ☐ Celery ☐ Lettuce
☐ Beet Greens ☐ Chicory ☐ Radish
☐ Cabbage ☐ Cucumber ☐ Tomato
☐ Chard ☐ Fennel ☐ Spinach

Bread -
☐ Melba Toast ☐ Melba Rounds ☐ Grissini

Fruit -

Dinner
(Choose one from each category)

Protein -
☐ Chicken
☐ Beef ☐ Seafood

Vegetable -
☐ Asparagus ☐ Celery ☐ Lettuce
☐ Beet Greens ☐ Chicory ☐ Radish
☐ Cabbage ☐ Cucumber ☐ Tomato
☐ Chard ☐ Fennel ☐ Spinach

Bread -
☐ Melba Toast ☐ Melba Rounds ☐ Grissini

Fruit -

Count your water here!

(2 liters or eight 8oz. glass recommended)

Comments for Today _____

_____

_____

_____

_____

TIP of the DAY
Take your measurements! It is fun to see those numbers go down as well!

Day 28

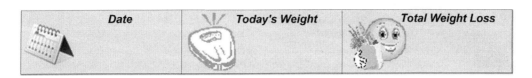

Date	Today's Weight	Total Weight Loss

Breakfast -- stay full drinking any amount of tea, coffee, or water.
(it all counts towards your total water for the day.)

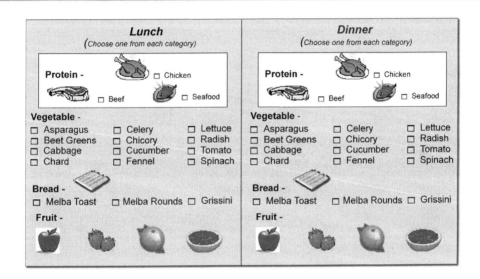

Lunch
(Choose one from each category)

Protein -
☐ Chicken
☐ Beef
☐ Seafood

Vegetable -
☐ Asparagus ☐ Celery ☐ Lettuce
☐ Beet Greens ☐ Chicory ☐ Radish
☐ Cabbage ☐ Cucumber ☐ Tomato
☐ Chard ☐ Fennel ☐ Spinach

Bread -
☐ Melba Toast ☐ Melba Rounds ☐ Grissini

Fruit -

Dinner
(Choose one from each category)

Protein -
☐ Chicken
☐ Beef
☐ Seafood

Vegetable -
☐ Asparagus ☐ Celery ☐ Lettuce
☐ Beet Greens ☐ Chicory ☐ Radish
☐ Cabbage ☐ Cucumber ☐ Tomato
☐ Chard ☐ Fennel ☐ Spinach

Bread -
☐ Melba Toast ☐ Melba Rounds ☐ Grissini

Fruit -

Count your water here!

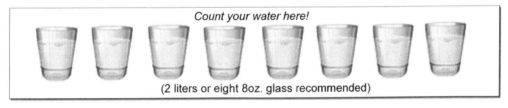

(2 liters or eight 8oz. glass recommended)

Comments for Today

TIP of the DAY
If you have a day or two of no weight loss, don't sweat it! Sometimes that happens, but it usually follows with a sudden big weight loss. Be patient!

Day 29

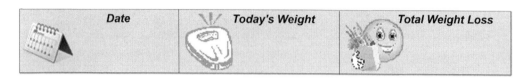

Date	Today's Weight	Total Weight Loss

Breakfast -- stay full drinking any amount of tea, coffee, or water.
(it all counts towards your total water for the day.)

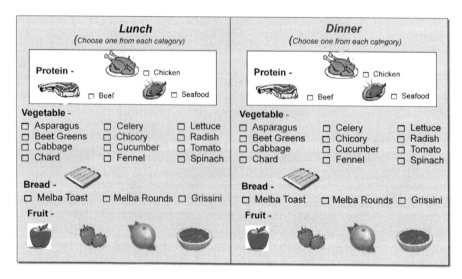

Lunch
(Choose one from each category)

Protein -
☐ Chicken
☐ Beef
☐ Seafood

Vegetable -
☐ Asparagus ☐ Celery ☐ Lettuce
☐ Beet Greens ☐ Chicory ☐ Radish
☐ Cabbage ☐ Cucumber ☐ Tomato
☐ Chard ☐ Fennel ☐ Spinach

Bread -
☐ Melba Toast ☐ Melba Rounds ☐ Grissini

Fruit -

Dinner
(Choose one from each category)

Protein -
☐ Chicken
☐ Beef
☐ Seafood

Vegetable -
☐ Asparagus ☐ Celery ☐ Lettuce
☐ Beet Greens ☐ Chicory ☐ Radish
☐ Cabbage ☐ Cucumber ☐ Tomato
☐ Chard ☐ Fennel ☐ Spinach

Bread -
☐ Melba Toast ☐ Melba Rounds ☐ Grissini

Fruit -

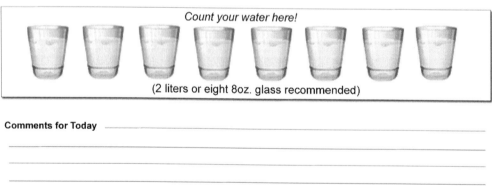

Count your water here!

(2 liters or eight 8oz. glass recommended)

Comments for Today

TIP of the DAY

Don't cheat! But if you do, take Cheaters Relief! It will help to make it less of a cheat. I don't want to encourage cheating but it would be better to already have this on hand for when that time comes. Available at www.myhcgsource.com.

Day 30

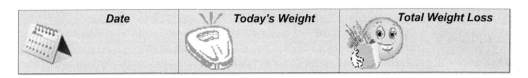

Date	Today's Weight	Total Weight Loss

Breakfast -- stay full drinking any amount of tea, coffee, or water.
(it all counts towards your total water for the day.)

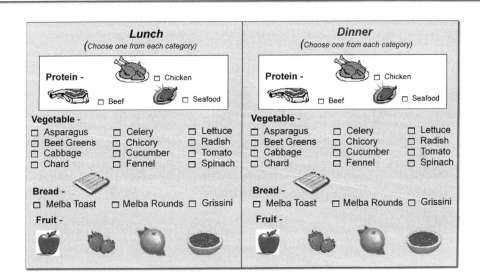

Lunch
(Choose one from each category)

Protein -
☐ Chicken
☐ Beef
☐ Seafood

Vegetable -
☐ Asparagus ☐ Celery ☐ Lettuce
☐ Beet Greens ☐ Chicory ☐ Radish
☐ Cabbage ☐ Cucumber ☐ Tomato
☐ Chard ☐ Fennel ☐ Spinach

Bread -
☐ Melba Toast ☐ Melba Rounds ☐ Grissini

Fruit -

Dinner
(Choose one from each category)

Protein -
☐ Chicken
☐ Beef
☐ Seafood

Vegetable -
☐ Asparagus ☐ Celery ☐ Lettuce
☐ Beet Greens ☐ Chicory ☐ Radish
☐ Cabbage ☐ Cucumber ☐ Tomato
☐ Chard ☐ Fennel ☐ Spinach

Bread -
☐ Melba Toast ☐ Melba Rounds ☐ Grissini

Fruit -

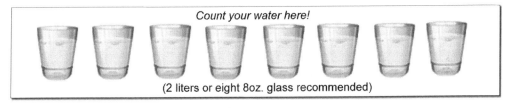

Count your water here!

(2 liters or eight 8oz. glass recommended)

Comments for Today

TIP of the DAY
Don't just cook these healthy meals for yourself! Make enough for the whole family! Why should you have to watch them pig out while you eat healthy? They can benefit from healthy cooking too!

Day 31

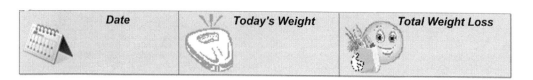

Date	Today's Weight	Total Weight Loss

Breakfast -- stay full drinking any amount of tea, coffee, or water.
(it all counts towards your total water for the day.)

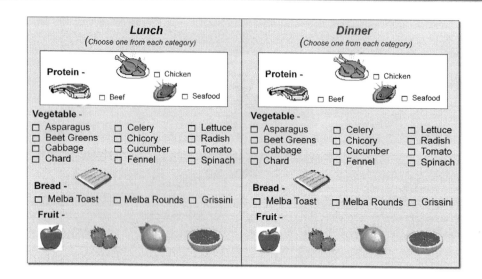

Lunch
(Choose one from each category)

Protein -
☐ Chicken
☐ Beef
☐ Seafood

Vegetable -
☐ Asparagus ☐ Celery ☐ Lettuce
☐ Beet Greens ☐ Chicory ☐ Radish
☐ Cabbage ☐ Cucumber ☐ Tomato
☐ Chard ☐ Fennel ☐ Spinach

Bread -
☐ Melba Toast ☐ Melba Rounds ☐ Grissini

Fruit -

Dinner
(Choose one from each category)

Protein -
☐ Chicken
☐ Beef
☐ Seafood

Vegetable -
☐ Asparagus ☐ Celery ☐ Lettuce
☐ Beet Greens ☐ Chicory ☐ Radish
☐ Cabbage ☐ Cucumber ☐ Tomato
☐ Chard ☐ Fennel ☐ Spinach

Bread -
☐ Melba Toast ☐ Melba Rounds ☐ Grissini

Fruit -

Count your water here!

(2 liters or eight 8oz. glass recommended)

Comments for Today

TIP of the DAY
Make your last fruit of the day into a dessert! Throw some strawberries, ice and vanilla cream stevia into a blender to make a frozen dessert! Try it with an orange too! Yummy! This is a great lifestyle change to keep for the rest of your life!

Day 32

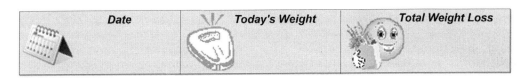

Date	Today's Weight	Total Weight Loss

Breakfast -- stay full drinking any amount of tea, coffee, or water.
(it all counts towards your total water for the day.)

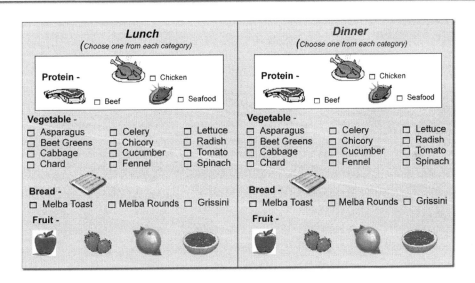

Lunch
(Choose one from each category)

Protein -
☐ Chicken
☐ Beef
☐ Seafood

Vegetable -
☐ Asparagus   ☐ Celery   ☐ Lettuce
☐ Beet Greens   ☐ Chicory   ☐ Radish
☐ Cabbage   ☐ Cucumber   ☐ Tomato
☐ Chard   ☐ Fennel   ☐ Spinach

Bread -
☐ Melba Toast   ☐ Melba Rounds   ☐ Grissini

Fruit -

Dinner
(Choose one from each category)

Protein -
☐ Chicken
☐ Beef
☐ Seafood

Vegetable -
☐ Asparagus   ☐ Celery   ☐ Lettuce
☐ Beet Greens   ☐ Chicory   ☐ Radish
☐ Cabbage   ☐ Cucumber   ☐ Tomato
☐ Chard   ☐ Fennel   ☐ Spinach

Bread -
☐ Melba Toast   ☐ Melba Rounds   ☐ Grissini

Fruit -

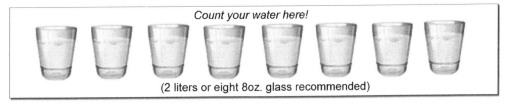

Count your water here!

(2 liters or eight 8oz. glass recommended)

Comments for Today _____

_____

_____

_____

_____

_____

TIP of the DAY
Make sure you are taking your HCG a half hour before you eat a meal.

Day 33

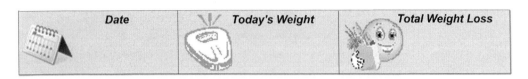

Date	Today's Weight	Total Weight Loss

Breakfast -- stay full drinking any amount of tea, coffee, or water.
(it all counts towards your total water for the day.)

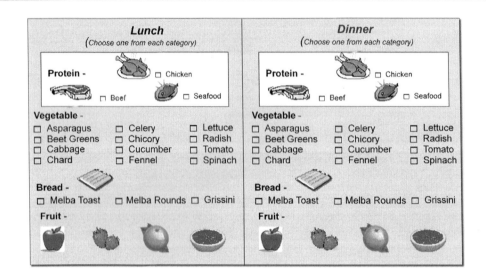

Lunch
(Choose one from each category)

Protein -
☐ Chicken
☐ Beef
☐ Seafood

Vegetable -
☐ Asparagus ☐ Celery ☐ Lettuce
☐ Beet Greens ☐ Chicory ☐ Radish
☐ Cabbage ☐ Cucumber ☐ Tomato
☐ Chard ☐ Fennel ☐ Spinach

Bread -
☐ Melba Toast ☐ Melba Rounds ☐ Grissini

Fruit -

Dinner
(Choose one from each category)

Protein -
☐ Chicken
☐ Beef
☐ Seafood

Vegetable -
☐ Asparagus ☐ Celery ☐ Lettuce
☐ Beet Greens ☐ Chicory ☐ Radish
☐ Cabbage ☐ Cucumber ☐ Tomato
☐ Chard ☐ Fennel ☐ Spinach

Bread -
☐ Melba Toast ☐ Melba Rounds ☐ Grissini

Fruit -

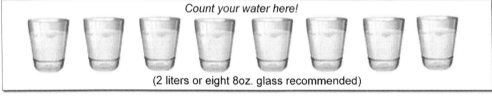

Count your water here!

(2 liters or eight 8oz. glass recommended)

Comments for Today _____

_____

_____

_____

_____

TIP of the DAY

Tell your friends about the diet! The more fellow dieters the more fun it is!

Day 34

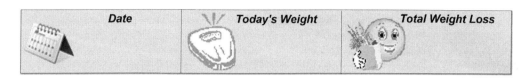

Date	Today's Weight	Total Weight Loss

Breakfast -- stay full drinking any amount of tea, coffee, or water.
(it all counts towards your total water for the day.)

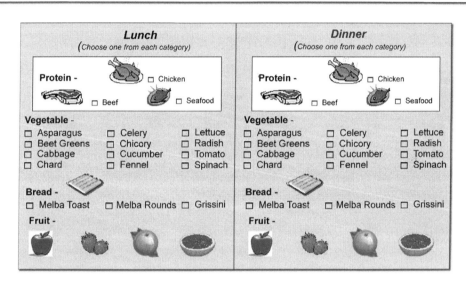

Lunch
(Choose one from each category)

Protein -
☐ Chicken
☐ Beef
☐ Seafood

Vegetable -
☐ Asparagus ☐ Celery ☐ Lettuce
☐ Beet Greens ☐ Chicory ☐ Radish
☐ Cabbage ☐ Cucumber ☐ Tomato
☐ Chard ☐ Fennel ☐ Spinach

Bread -
☐ Melba Toast ☐ Melba Rounds ☐ Grissini

Fruit -

Dinner
(Choose one from each category)

Protein -
☐ Chicken
☐ Beef
☐ Seafood

Vegetable -
☐ Asparagus ☐ Celery ☐ Lettuce
☐ Beet Greens ☐ Chicory ☐ Radish
☐ Cabbage ☐ Cucumber ☐ Tomato
☐ Chard ☐ Fennel ☐ Spinach

Bread -
☐ Melba Toast ☐ Melba Rounds ☐ Grissini

Fruit -

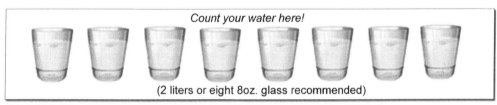

Count your water here!

(2 liters or eight 8oz. glass recommended)

Comments for Today

TIP of the DAY
Do not drink or brush your teeth for 15 minutes before or after taking your HCG.

Day 35

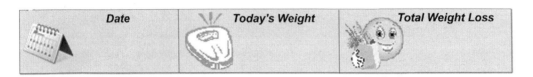

Date	Today's Weight	Total Weight Loss

Breakfast -- stay full drinking any amount of tea, coffee, or water.
(it all counts towards your total water for the day.)

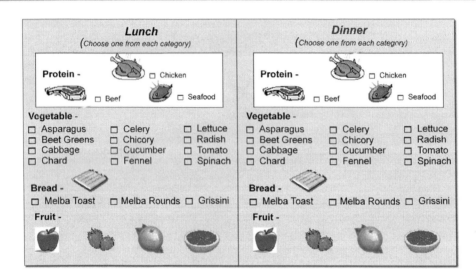

Lunch
(Choose one from each category)

Protein -
□ Chicken
□ Beef
□ Seafood

Vegetable -
□ Asparagus   □ Celery   □ Lettuce
□ Beet Greens □ Chicory □ Radish
□ Cabbage   □ Cucumber □ Tomato
□ Chard   □ Fennel   □ Spinach

Bread -
□ Melba Toast   □ Melba Rounds   □ Grissini

Fruit -

Dinner
(Choose one from each category)

Protein -
□ Chicken
□ Beef
□ Seafood

Vegetable -
□ Asparagus   □ Celery   □ Lettuce
□ Beet Greens □ Chicory □ Radish
□ Cabbage   □ Cucumber □ Tomato
□ Chard   □ Fennel   □ Spinach

Bread -
□ Melba Toast   □ Melba Rounds   □ Grissini

Fruit -

Count your water here!

(2 liters or eight 8oz. glass recommended)

Comments for Today

TIP of the DAY

Try a new vegetable. Maybe you have never cooked with fennel or mustard greens!

Day 36

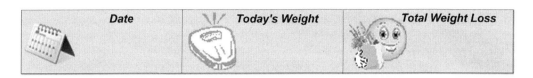

	Date	Today's Weight	Total Weight Loss

Breakfast -- stay full drinking any amount of tea, coffee, or water.
(it all counts towards your total water for the day.)

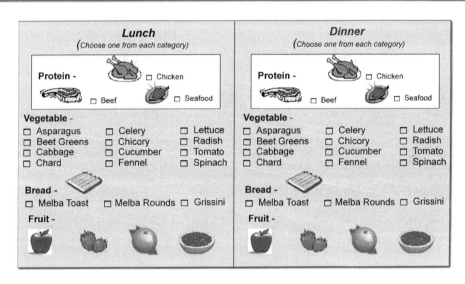

Lunch
(Choose one from each category)

Protein -
☐ Chicken
☐ Beef
☐ Seafood

Vegetable -
☐ Asparagus ☐ Celery ☐ Lettuce
☐ Beet Greens ☐ Chicory ☐ Radish
☐ Cabbage ☐ Cucumber ☐ Tomato
☐ Chard ☐ Fennel ☐ Spinach

Bread -
☐ Melba Toast ☐ Melba Rounds ☐ Grissini

Fruit -

Dinner
(Choose one from each category)

Protein -
☐ Chicken
☐ Beef
☐ Seafood

Vegetable -
☐ Asparagus ☐ Celery ☐ Lettuce
☐ Beet Greens ☐ Chicory ☐ Radish
☐ Cabbage ☐ Cucumber ☐ Tomato
☐ Chard ☐ Fennel ☐ Spinach

Bread -
☐ Melba Toast ☐ Melba Rounds ☐ Grissini

Fruit -

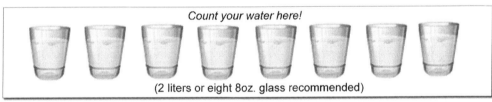

Count your water here!

(2 liters or eight 8oz. glass recommended)

Comments for Today

TIP of the DAY

If you are a coffee drinker and can't do without cream, why not try something new? Try drinking hot tea with stevia for a change.

Day 37

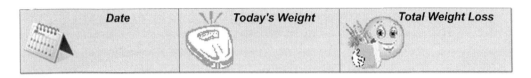

Date	Today's Weight	Total Weight Loss

Breakfast -- stay full drinking any amount of tea, coffee, or water.
(it all counts towards your total water for the day.)

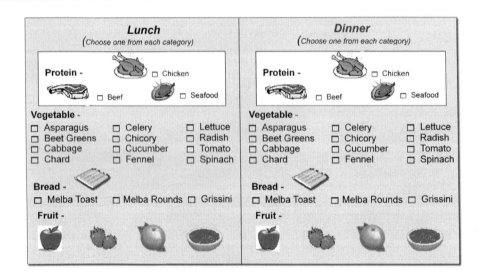

Lunch	**Dinner**
(Choose one from each category)	(Choose one from each category)

Lunch
(Choose one from each category)

Protein -
☐ Chicken
☐ Beef   ☐ Seafood

Vegetable -
☐ Asparagus   ☐ Celery   ☐ Lettuce
☐ Beet Greens ☐ Chicory   ☐ Radish
☐ Cabbage   ☐ Cucumber   ☐ Tomato
☐ Chard   ☐ Fennel   ☐ Spinach

Bread -
☐ Melba Toast   ☐ Melba Rounds ☐ Grissini

Fruit -

Dinner
(Choose one from each category)

Protein -
☐ Chicken
☐ Beef   ☐ Seafood

Vegetable -
☐ Asparagus   ☐ Celery   ☐ Lettuce
☐ Beet Greens ☐ Chicory   ☐ Radish
☐ Cabbage   ☐ Cucumber   ☐ Tomato
☐ Chard   ☐ Fennel   ☐ Spinach

Bread -
☐ Melba Toast   ☐ Melba Rounds ☐ Grissini

Fruit -

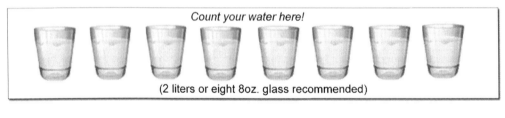

Count your water here!

(2 liters or eight 8oz. glass recommended)

Comments for Today

TIP of the DAY

Feel your belly! It's amazing how much it goes down from eating smaller quantities!

Day 38

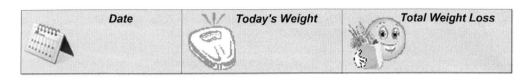

Date	Today's Weight	Total Weight Loss

Breakfast -- stay full drinking any amount of tea, coffee, or water.
(it all counts towards your total water for the day.)

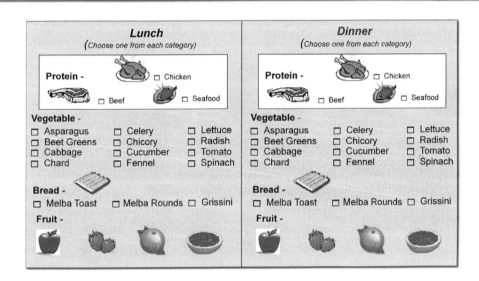

Lunch
(*Choose one from each category*)

Protein -
☐ Chicken
☐ Beef
☐ Seafood

Vegetable -
☐ Asparagus ☐ Celery ☐ Lettuce
☐ Beet Greens ☐ Chicory ☐ Radish
☐ Cabbage ☐ Cucumber ☐ Tomato
☐ Chard ☐ Fennel ☐ Spinach

Bread -
☐ Melba Toast ☐ Melba Rounds ☐ Grissini

Fruit -

Dinner
(*Choose one from each category*)

Protein -
☐ Chicken
☐ Beef
☐ Seafood

Vegetable -
☐ Asparagus ☐ Celery ☐ Lettuce
☐ Beet Greens ☐ Chicory ☐ Radish
☐ Cabbage ☐ Cucumber ☐ Tomato
☐ Chard ☐ Fennel ☐ Spinach

Bread -
☐ Melba Toast ☐ Melba Rounds ☐ Grissini

Fruit -

Count your water here!

(2 liters or eight 8oz. glass recommended)

Comments for Today

TIP of the DAY
Take pride that you are in control of your appetite! Don't look at non-dieters with envy! Think of them as out-of-control!

Day 39

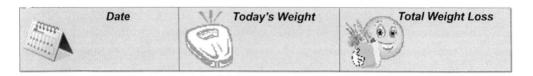

Date	Today's Weight	Total Weight Loss

Breakfast -- stay full drinking any amount of tea, coffee, or water.
(it all counts towards your total water for the day.)

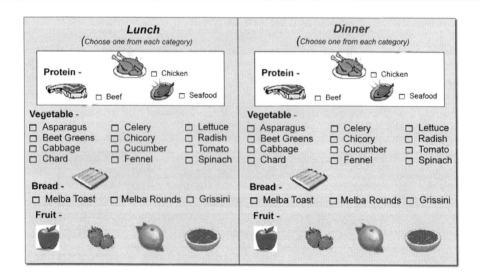

Lunch
(Choose one from each category)

Protein -
☐ Chicken
☐ Beef
☐ Seafood

Vegetable -
☐ Asparagus   ☐ Celery   ☐ Lettuce
☐ Beet Greens ☐ Chicory   ☐ Radish
☐ Cabbage   ☐ Cucumber ☐ Tomato
☐ Chard   ☐ Fennel   ☐ Spinach

Bread -
☐ Melba Toast   ☐ Melba Rounds ☐ Grissini

Fruit -

Dinner
(Choose one from each category)

Protein -
☐ Chicken
☐ Beef
☐ Seafood

Vegetable -
☐ Asparagus   ☐ Celery   ☐ Lettuce
☐ Beet Greens ☐ Chicory   ☐ Radish
☐ Cabbage   ☐ Cucumber ☐ Tomato
☐ Chard   ☐ Fennel   ☐ Spinach

Bread -
☐ Melba Toast   ☐ Melba Rounds ☐ Grissini

Fruit -

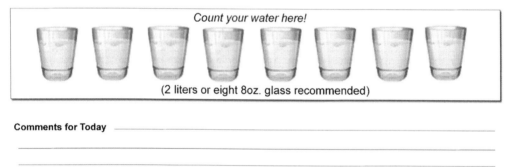

Count your water here!

(2 liters or eight 8oz. glass recommended)

Comments for Today

TIP of the DAY

If your weight loss is stalled, try eating fish or chicken for a while and stay away from beef.

Day 40

(Last day on HCG)

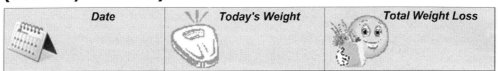

Date	Today's Weight	Total Weight Loss

Breakfast -- stay full drinking any amount of tea, coffee, or water.
(it all counts towards your total water for the day.)

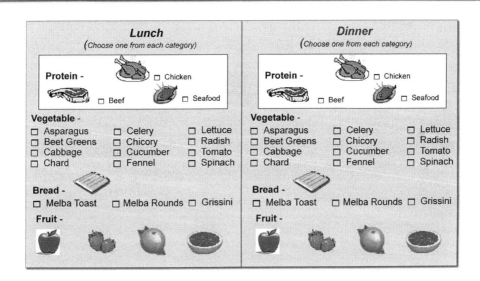

Lunch
(Choose one from each category)

Protein - □ Chicken
□ Beef □ Seafood

Vegetable -
□ Asparagus □ Celery □ Lettuce
□ Beet Greens □ Chicory □ Radish
□ Cabbage □ Cucumber □ Tomato
□ Chard □ Fennel □ Spinach

Bread -
□ Melba Toast □ Melba Rounds □ Grissini

Fruit -

Dinner
(Choose one from each category)

Protein - □ Chicken
□ Beef □ Seafood

Vegetable -
□ Asparagus □ Celery □ Lettuce
□ Beet Greens □ Chicory □ Radish
□ Cabbage □ Cucumber □ Tomato
□ Chard □ Fennel □ Spinach

Bread -
□ Melba Toast □ Melba Rounds □ Grissini

Fruit -

Count your water here!

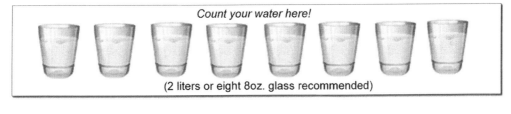

(2 liters or eight 8oz. glass recommended)

Comments for Today _____

TIP of the DAY
If you are having headaches, you may need to take a potassium supplement. Headaches can be a sign of low potassium.

Day 41

(No HCG)

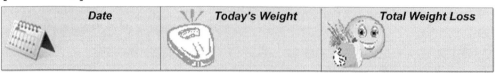

Date	Today's Weight	Total Weight Loss

Breakfast -- stay full drinking any amount of tea, coffee, or water.
(it all counts towards your total water for the day.)

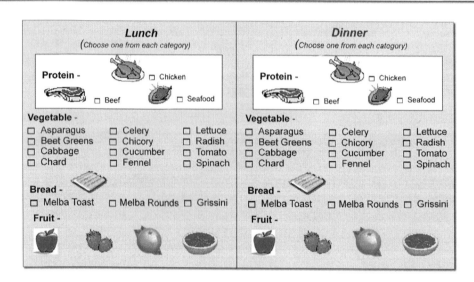

Lunch
(*Choose one from each category*)

Protein -
- ☐ Chicken
- ☐ Beef
- ☐ Seafood

Vegetable -
- ☐ Asparagus
- ☐ Beet Greens
- ☐ Cabbage
- ☐ Chard
- ☐ Celery
- ☐ Chicory
- ☐ Cucumber
- ☐ Fennel
- ☐ Lettuce
- ☐ Radish
- ☐ Tomato
- ☐ Spinach

Bread -
- ☐ Melba Toast
- ☐ Melba Rounds
- ☐ Grissini

Fruit -

Dinner
(*Choose one from each category*)

Protein -
- ☐ Chicken
- ☐ Beef
- ☐ Seafood

Vegetable -
- ☐ Asparagus
- ☐ Beet Greens
- ☐ Cabbage
- ☐ Chard
- ☐ Celery
- ☐ Chicory
- ☐ Cucumber
- ☐ Fennel
- ☐ Lettuce
- ☐ Radish
- ☐ Tomato
- ☐ Spinach

Bread -
- ☐ Melba Toast
- ☐ Melba Rounds
- ☐ Grissini

Fruit -

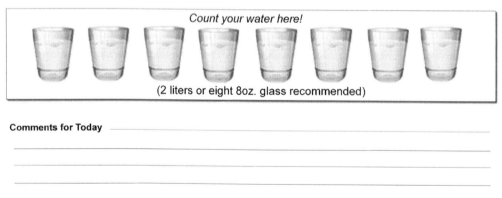

Count your water here!

(2 liters or eight 8oz. glass recommended)

Comments for Today _____

_____

_____

_____

_____

TIP of the DAY

Have a plan for Phase 3 Maintenance. If you are planning to pig out after phase 2, you will gain the weight back! You must follow the Maintenance plan for a full 3 weeks to lock in this weight loss and reset your hypothalamus.

Day 42

(No HCG)

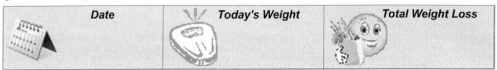

Date	Today's Weight	Total Weight Loss

Breakfast -- stay full drinking any amount of tea, coffee, or water.
(it all counts towards your total water for the day.)

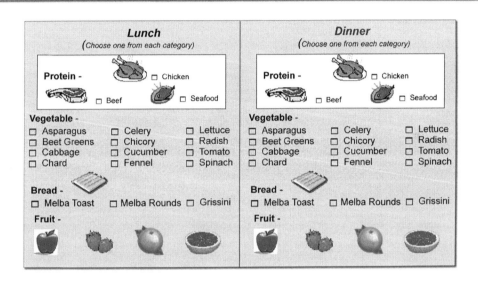

Lunch
(Choose one from each category)

Protein -
☐ Chicken
☐ Beef
☐ Seafood

Vegetable -
☐ Asparagus ☐ Celery ☐ Lettuce
☐ Beet Greens ☐ Chicory ☐ Radish
☐ Cabbage ☐ Cucumber ☐ Tomato
☐ Chard ☐ Fennel ☐ Spinach

Bread -
☐ Melba Toast ☐ Melba Rounds ☐ Grissini

Fruit -

Dinner
(Choose one from each category)

Protein -
☐ Chicken
☐ Beef
☐ Seafood

Vegetable -
☐ Asparagus ☐ Celery ☐ Lettuce
☐ Beet Greens ☐ Chicory ☐ Radish
☐ Cabbage ☐ Cucumber ☐ Tomato
☐ Chard ☐ Fennel ☐ Spinach

Bread -
☐ Melba Toast ☐ Melba Rounds ☐ Grissini

Fruit -

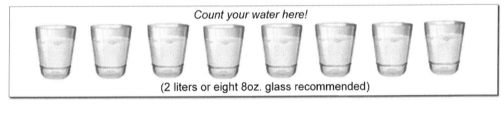

Count your water here!

(2 liters or eight 8oz. glass recommended)

Comments for Today

TIP of the DAY

If you are starting to feel hunger without the HCG pumping through your body anymore, feel free to add 2 eggs to tomorrow's breakfast.

Day 43

(Last Day of 500 Calorie Diet!)
(No HCG)

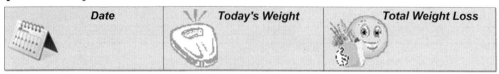

Date	Today's Weight	Total Weight Loss

Breakfast -- stay full drinking any amount of tea, coffee, or water.
(it all counts towards your total water for the day.)

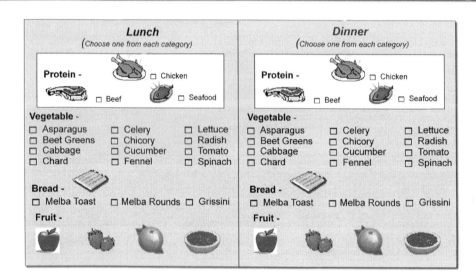

Lunch
(Choose one from each category)

Protein -
- ☐ Chicken
- ☐ Beef
- ☐ Seafood

Vegetable -
- ☐ Asparagus ☐ Celery ☐ Lettuce
- ☐ Beet Greens ☐ Chicory ☐ Radish
- ☐ Cabbage ☐ Cucumber ☐ Tomato
- ☐ Chard ☐ Fennel ☐ Spinach

Bread -
- ☐ Melba Toast ☐ Melba Rounds ☐ Grissini

Fruit -

Dinner
(Choose one from each category)

Protein -
- ☐ Chicken
- ☐ Beef
- ☐ Seafood

Vegetable -
- ☐ Asparagus ☐ Celery ☐ Lettuce
- ☐ Beet Greens ☐ Chicory ☐ Radish
- ☐ Cabbage ☐ Cucumber ☐ Tomato
- ☐ Chard ☐ Fennel ☐ Spinach

Bread -
- ☐ Melba Toast ☐ Melba Rounds ☐ Grissini

Fruit -

Count your water here!

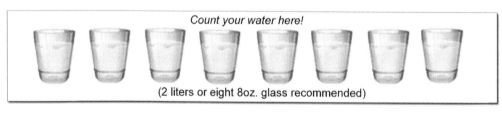

(2 liters or eight 8oz. glass recommended)

Comments for Today

TIP of the DAY
Blog about your success or your struggles with fellow HCG dieters at www.myhcgsource.com.

Maintenance Part 1

Once you've taken off 20 or 30 pounds you should look and feel better than you have in years. At this point many of you will be interested in maintaining your weight loss. This is when the rest of the HCG diet comes into play. Phase 3 helps you keep off the pounds.

Phase 3 - Maintenance

To maintain your weight loss you must reset the set-point that helps govern your day-to-day weight. If you want to do this you will need to stick to the 500-calories-per-day diet for 3 extra days—without the HCG. When the 3 days are over the HCG will have left your body.

Over the next 3 weeks you must continue avoiding all sugar and starches, but otherwise you can eat almost anything. You will be eating about 2,000 calories per day, more if you work out or regularly play sports. The object is to stay within 2 pounds of your weight at the end of Phase 2. If you exceed the 2-pound limit, follow the following regimen for a day: no breakfast or lunch, but plenty of fat-and-sugar-free liquids, then for dinner a huge steak with either an apple or a raw tomato. That should take off the excess weight, and you can return to the 2,000-calorie diet. If you should lose more than 2 pounds from your last HCG weight, you need to eat more.

Those who gain all their weight back are usually the people who never progressed to Phase 3. The Phase 2 VLCD is designed to take off the pounds. Though it quadruples your caloric intake, Phase 3 keeps the pounds off. The Phase 3 regimen helps retrain your body to accept and maintain this new weight.

Maintenance Day 1

Eat what you want, just NO Sugar, NO Starch!

Today I ate _____

_____

_____

_____

_____

_____

_____

_____ _____

I probably shouldn't have ate_____

_____

_____

Today's Weight

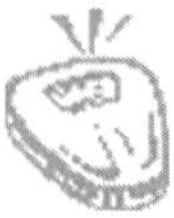

**Are you within 2 lbs.
of your last HCG Weight?**

YES   NO

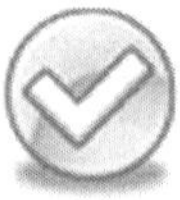

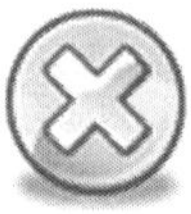

Maintenance Day 2

Eat what you want, just NO Sugar, NO Starch!

Today I ate _____

_____

_____

_____

_____

_____

_____

I probably shouldn't have ate_____

_____

_____

Today's Weight

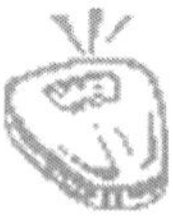

**Are you within 2 lbs.
of your last HCG Weight?**

YES   NO

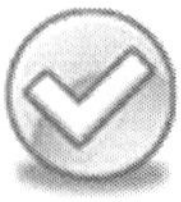

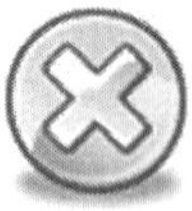

Maintenance Day 3

Eat what you want, just NO Sugar, NO Starch!

Today I ate _____
_____
_____
_____
_____
_____
_____
_____

I probably shouldn't have ate_____
_____
_____

Today's Weight

**Are you within 2 lbs.
of your last HCG Weight?**

YES   NO

Maintenance Day 4

Eat what you want, just NO Sugar, NO Starch!

Today I ate _____
_____
_____
_____
_____
_____
_____

I probably shouldn't have ate_____
_____
_____

Today's Weight

**Are you within 2 lbs.
of your last HCG Weight?**

YES   NO

Maintenance Day 5

Eat what you want, just NO Sugar, NO Starch!

Today I ate _____

_____

_____

_____

_____

_____

_____

I probably shouldn't have ate_____

_____

_____

Today's Weight

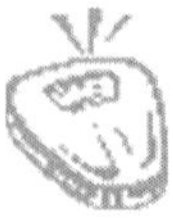

Are you within 2 lbs. of your last HCG Weight?

YES   NO

Maintenance Day 6

Eat what you want, just NO Sugar, NO Starch!

Today I ate _____

_____

_____

_____

_____

_____

_____

I probably shouldn't have ate_____

_____

_____

Today's Weight

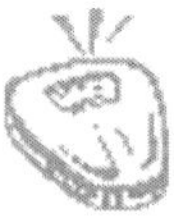

Are you within 2 lbs. of your last HCG Weight?

YES   NO

Maintenance Day 7

Eat what you want, just NO Sugar, NO Starch!

Today I ate _____
_____
_____
_____
_____
_____
_____
_____

I probably shouldn't have ate_____
_____
_____

Today's Weight

Are you within 2 lbs. of your last HCG Weight?

YES   NO

Maintenance Day 8

Eat what you want, just NO Sugar, NO Starch!

Today I ate _____
_____
_____
_____
_____
_____
_____
_____

I probably shouldn't have ate_____
_____
_____

Today's Weight

Are you within 2 lbs. of your last HCG Weight?

YES   NO

Maintenance Day 9

Eat what you want, just NO Sugar, NO Starch!

Today I ate _____

_____

_____

_____

_____

_____

_____

I probably shouldn't have ate_____

_____

_____

Today's Weight

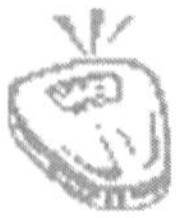

**Are you within 2 lbs.
of your last HCG Weight?**

YES   NO

Maintenance Day 10

Eat what you want, just NO Sugar, NO Starch!

Today I ate _____

_____

_____

_____

_____

_____

_____

I probably shouldn't have ate_____

_____

_____

Today's Weight

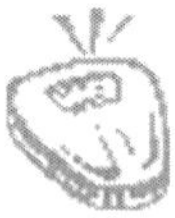

**Are you within 2 lbs.
of your last HCG Weight?**

YES   NO

Maintenance Day 11

Eat what you want, just NO Sugar, NO Starch!

Today I ate _____

_____

_____

_____

_____

_____

_____

I probably shouldn't have ate_____

_____

_____

Today's Weight

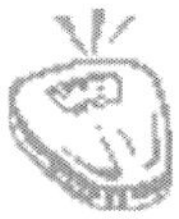

**Are you within 2 lbs.
of your last HCG Weight?**

YES   NO

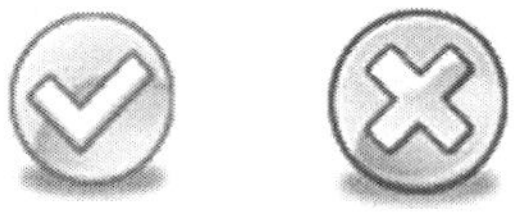

Maintenance Day 12

Eat what you want, just NO Sugar, NO Starch!

Today I ate _____

_____

_____

_____

_____

_____

_____

I probably shouldn't have ate_____

_____

_____

Today's Weight

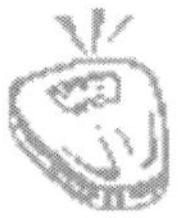

**Are you within 2 lbs.
of your last HCG Weight?**

YES   NO

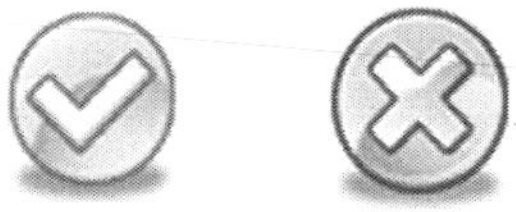

Maintenance Day 13

Eat what you want, just NO Sugar, NO Starch!

Today I ate _____

_____

_____

_____

_____

_____

_____

I probably shouldn't have ate_____

_____

_____

Today's Weight

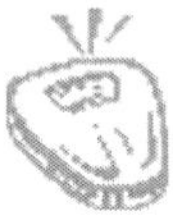

**Are you within 2 lbs.
of your last HCG Weight?**

YES | NO

Maintenance Day 14

Eat what you want, just NO Sugar, NO Starch!

Today I ate _____

_____

_____

_____

_____

_____

_____

I probably shouldn't have ate_____

_____

_____

Today's Weight

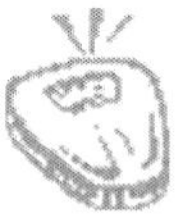

**Are you within 2 lbs.
of your last HCG Weight?**

YES | NO

Maintenance Day 15

Eat what you want, just NO Sugar, NO Starch!

Today I ate _____

_____

_____

_____

_____

_____

_____

_____

I probably shouldn't have ate_____

_____

_____

Today's Weight

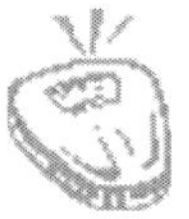

Are you within 2 lbs.
of your last HCG Weight?

YES   NO

Maintenance Day 16

Eat what you want, just NO Sugar, NO Starch!

Today I ate _____

_____

_____

_____

_____

_____

_____

I probably shouldn't have ate_____

_____

_____

Today's Weight

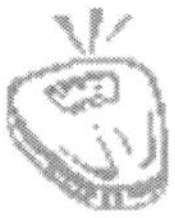

Are you within 2 lbs.
of your last HCG Weight?

YES   NO

Maintenance Day 17

Eat what you want, just NO Sugar, NO Starch!

Today I ate _____
_____
_____
_____
_____
_____
_____
_____

I probably shouldn't have ate_____
_____
_____

Today's Weight

Are you within 2 lbs. of your last HCG Weight?

YES   NO

Maintenance Day 18

Eat what you want, just NO Sugar, NO Starch!

Today I ate _____
_____
_____
_____
_____
_____
_____

I probably shouldn't have ate_____
_____
_____

Today's Weight

Are you within 2 lbs. of your last HCG Weight?

YES   NO

Maintenance Day 19

Eat what you want, just NO Sugar, NO Starch!

Today I ate _____
_____
_____
_____
_____
_____
_____
_____

I probably shouldn't have ate_____
_____
_____

Today's Weight

**Are you within 2 lbs.
of your last HCG Weight?**

YES   NO

Maintenance Day 20

Eat what you want, just NO Sugar, NO Starch!

Today I ate _____
_____
_____
_____
_____
_____
_____

I probably shouldn't have ate_____
_____
_____

Today's Weight

**Are you within 2 lbs.
of your last HCG Weight?**

YES   NO

Maintenance Day 21

Eat what you want, just NO Sugar, NO Starch!

Today I ate _____
_____
_____
_____
_____
_____
_____
_____

I probably shouldn't have ate_____
_____
_____

Today's Weight

Are you within 2 lbs. of your last HCG Weight?

YES   NO

Maintenance Part 2

Good job! Well Done! You have now finished with 3 full weeks of Maintenance! All in all, you are probably pretty impressed with your weight loss! If you have had trouble maintaining your weight loss and have gained some back, why not look back at this log book and figure out where you might have missed the mark. Hopefully, you were able to compensate for any gain by doing a "steak day". That usually will do the trick to get you back on track!

If you have reached your goal, congratulations! Now is the time to work towards a healthy lifestyle. You are now permitted to start adding starches and sugars back into your diet. Be careful and do this slowly! Do not revert back to your previous way of eating! You have a new lease on life, so to say. Don't blow it! Sure you can enjoy some of your favorite foods, but do so with moderation. You probably noticed that it doesn't take as much to fill your stomach anymore and that is a good thing! Let's keep it that way! Continue tracking your food intake on the following pages, just to make sure that you get a good start on your new healthy lifestyle. You don't have to keep tracking for the rest of your life. But start on your way, with controlled eating so that you are aware of how your body responds to the foods you are eating. Make sure to incorporate exercise into your life as well, so that you will live long and prosper!

If you have more weight to lose, you need to wait until day 42 of Maintenance until you are cleared to do the HCG diet again. You are welcome to do as many rounds of this diet as you need to accomplish your goals. Just make sure that you have a full 42 days of not taking any HCG before you resume using the product again. This will ensure that the HCG will work just as effectively each time you choose to do this diet. Remember, HCG is like having an ace up your sleeve! It's your secret weapon that allows you to survive on a very low calorie diet without suffering hunger pains! Don't ruin it for yourself by rushing or skipping the Maintenance phase of this diet.

Maintenance Day 22

SLOWLY add sugar and starch!

Today I ate _____

_____

_____

_____

_____

_____

_____

I probably shouldn't have ate_____

_____

_____

Today's Weight

**Are you within 2 lbs.
of your last HCG Weight?**

YES   NO

Maintenance Day 23

SLOWLY add sugar and starch!

Today I ate _____

_____

_____

_____

_____

_____

_____

I probably shouldn't have ate_____

_____

_____

Today's Weight

**Are you within 2 lbs.
of your last HCG Weight?**

YES   NO

Maintenance Day 24

SLOWLY add sugar and starch!

Today I ate _____

_____

_____

_____

_____

_____

_____

I probably shouldn't have ate_____

_____

_____

Today's Weight

**Are you within 2 lbs.
of your last HCG Weight?**

YES   NO

Maintenance Day 25

SLOWLY add sugar and starch!

Today I ate _____

_____

_____

_____

_____

_____

_____

I probably shouldn't have ate_____

_____

_____

Today's Weight

**Are you within 2 lbs.
of your last HCG Weight?**

YES   NO

Maintenance Day 26

SLOWLY add sugar and starch!

Today I ate _____

_____

_____

_____

_____

_____

_____

I probably shouldn't have ate_____

_____

_____

Today's Weight

Are you within 2 lbs. of your last HCG Weight?

YES   NO

Maintenance Day 27

SLOWLY add sugar and starch!

Today I ate _____

_____

_____

_____

_____

_____

_____

I probably shouldn't have ate_____

_____

_____

Today's Weight

Are you within 2 lbs. of your last HCG Weight?

YES   NO

74

Maintenance Day 28

SLOWLY add sugar and starch!

Today I ate _____

_____

_____

_____

_____

_____

_____

I probably shouldn't have ate_____

_____

_____

Today's Weight

**Are you within 2 lbs.
of your last HCG Weight?**

YES   NO

Maintenance Day 29

SLOWLY add sugar and starch!

Today I ate _____

_____

_____

_____

_____

_____

_____

I probably shouldn't have ate_____

_____

_____

Today's Weight

**Are you within 2 lbs.
of your last HCG Weight?**

YES   NO

Maintenance Day 30

SLOWLY add sugar and starch!

Today I ate _____

_____

_____

_____

_____

_____

_____

I probably shouldn't have ate_____

_____

_____

Today's Weight

**Are you within 2 lbs.
of your last HCG Weight?**

YES   NO

Maintenance Day 31

SLOWLY add sugar and starch!

Today I ate _____

_____

_____

_____

_____

_____

_____

I probably shouldn't have ate_____

_____

_____

Today's Weight

**Are you within 2 lbs.
of your last HCG Weight?**

YES   NO

Maintenance Day 32

SLOWLY add sugar and starch!

Today I ate _____
_____
_____
_____
_____
_____
_____
_____

I probably shouldn't have ate_____
_____
_____

Today's Weight

Are you within 2 lbs. of your last HCG Weight?

YES   NO

Maintenance Day 33

SLOWLY add sugar and starch!

Today I ate _____
_____
_____
_____
_____
_____
_____

I probably shouldn't have ate_____
_____
_____

Today's Weight

Are you within 2 lbs. of your last HCG Weight?

YES   NO

Maintenance Day 34

SLOWLY add sugar and starch!

Today I ate _____

_____

_____

_____

_____

_____

_____

I probably shouldn't have ate_____ _____

_____

_____

Today's Weight

Are you within 2 lbs. of your last HCG Weight?

YES   NO

Maintenance Day 35

SLOWLY add sugar and starch!

Today I ate _____

_____

_____

_____

_____

_____

_____

I probably shouldn't have ate_____

_____

_____

Today's Weight

Are you within 2 lbs. of your last HCG Weight?

YES   NO

Maintenance Day 36

SLOWLY add sugar and starch!

Today I ate _____

_____

_____

_____

_____

_____

_____

_____

I probably shouldn't have ate_____

_____

_____

Today's Weight

**Are you within 2 lbs.
of your last HCG Weight?**

YES   NO

Maintenance Day 37

SLOWLY add sugar and starch!

Today I ate _____

_____

_____

_____

_____

_____

_____

I probably shouldn't have ate_____

_____

_____

Today's Weight

**Are you within 2 lbs.
of your last HCG Weight?**

YES   NO

Maintenance Day 38

SLOWLY add sugar and starch!

Today I ate _____

_____

_____

_____

_____

_____

_____

I probably shouldn't have ate_____ _____

_____

_____

Today's Weight

Are you within 2 lbs. of your last HCG Weight?

YES   NO

Maintenance Day 39

SLOWLY add sugar and starch!

Today I ate _____

_____

_____

_____

_____

_____

_____

I probably shouldn't have ate_____

_____

_____

Today's Weight

Are you within 2 lbs. of your last HCG Weight?

YES   NO

Maintenance Day 40

SLOWLY add sugar and starch!

Today I ate _____
_____
_____
_____
_____
_____
_____
_____

I probably shouldn't have ate_____
_____
_____

Today's Weight

**Are you within 2 lbs.
of your last HCG Weight?**

YES   NO

Maintenance Day 41

SLOWLY add sugar and starch!

Today I ate _____
_____
_____
_____
_____
_____
_____
_____

I probably shouldn't have ate_____
_____
_____

Today's Weight

**Are you within 2 lbs.
of your last HCG Weight?**

YES   NO

Maintenance Day 42

SLOWLY add sugar and starch!

Today I ate _____

_____

_____

_____

_____

_____

_____

I probably shouldn't have ate_____

_____

_____

Today's Weight

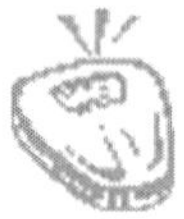

Are you within 2 lbs. of your last HCG Weight?

YES   NO

Ready to celebrate?!

O.K. Go ahead!!!!

You deserve it!

Then just as soon as you are done, come back

to your healthy eating, and start adding

physical activity into your daily life.

Remember, your goal is optimal health!

If you have more to lose,

let's do it again!